CONTENTS

CHAPTER 1: INTRODUCTION TO CHRONIC HIVES

Definition and Classification of Chronic Hives

Chronic hives, clinically termed as chronic idiopathic urticaria (CIU), is a perplexing dermatological condition characterized by the recurrent appearance of wheals or hives on the skin. These wheals are typically raised, red, and intensely itchy, varying in size and shape, and can occur anywhere on the body. Unlike acute urticaria, which resolves within six weeks, chronic hives persist for more than six weeks, often lasting months or even years. The term "idiopathic" denotes the absence of a known cause in the majority of cases, making the condition challenging to manage and understand fully.

Classification:

1. **Chronic Idiopathic Urticaria (CIU):** This subtype accounts for the majority of cases of chronic hives, where no identifiable trigger or underlying cause can be found despite thorough investigation. CIU is diagnosed based on the presence of recurrent wheals and/or angioedema for at least six weeks, with no obvious external cause.

2. **Chronic Spontaneous Urticaria (CSU):** CSU is a broader term encompassing chronic hives with known triggers or associated conditions. While CIU falls under this

umbrella, CSU also includes cases where specific triggers such as physical stimuli (e.g., pressure, cold, heat), infections, medications, or underlying systemic diseases (e.g., autoimmune disorders, thyroid dysfunction) are identified.

3. **Physical Urticaria:** This subtype refers to chronic hives triggered by physical stimuli such as pressure (dermatographic urticaria), cold (cold urticaria), heat (cholinergic urticaria), vibration, or sun exposure (solar urticaria). Physical urticarias may coexist with CIU or occur independently.

4. **Autoimmune Urticaria:** In a subset of chronic hives patients, autoimmune mechanisms are implicated, leading to the production of autoantibodies targeting mast cells or basophils. Autoimmune urticaria may present with features of CIU but is distinguished by the presence of specific autoantibodies detected through laboratory testing.

5. **Dermatographism:** Also known as dermatographic urticaria, this form of physical urticaria is characterized by the appearance of wheals in response to firm stroking or scratching of the skin. While dermatographism is typically considered a subtype of physical urticaria, it may also be present concurrently with CIU.

6. **Delayed Pressure Urticaria:** This rare subtype of physical urticaria is characterized by the delayed onset of wheals and swelling following sustained pressure on the skin, such as from tight clothing or prolonged sitting or standing.

Clinical Presentation:

Chronic hives typically present as erythematous, edematous wheals with surrounding erythema, often accompanied by intense pruritus (itching). The wheals may vary in size, shape, and distribution, appearing and disappearing spontaneously over hours to days. In severe cases, angioedema, characterized by deeper swelling in the dermis and subcutaneous tissues, may occur, particularly affecting the face, lips, eyelids, and extremities. Angioedema can be associated with significant discomfort and, in rare instances, poses a risk of airway compromise.

Differential Diagnosis:

The diagnosis of chronic hives requires careful consideration of other dermatological conditions presenting with similar features. Differential diagnoses include acute urticaria, urticarial vasculitis, angioedema without wheals, eczema, contact dermatitis, erythema multiforme, and drug eruptions. Differentiating between these conditions is crucial for appropriate management and treatment.

Conclusion:

In summary, chronic hives represent a heterogeneous group of dermatological disorders characterized by the recurrent appearance of wheals and/or angioedema lasting more than six weeks. While the majority of cases fall under the category of chronic idiopathic urticaria, various subtypes with known triggers or associated conditions exist, each requiring tailored management strategies. Understanding the classification and clinical presentation of chronic hives is essential for accurate diagnosis and effective treatment, thereby improving patients' quality of life.

Epidemiology of Chronic Hives

Understanding the epidemiology of chronic hives, also known as chronic idiopathic urticaria (CIU), is crucial for healthcare professionals to grasp the magnitude of the condition's impact on individuals and society as a whole. Epidemiological studies provide insights into the prevalence, incidence, risk factors, geographic variations, and demographic characteristics associated with chronic hives. By examining these factors, researchers and clinicians can better tailor prevention strategies, allocate resources effectively, and improve patient care.

Prevalence and Incidence:

Chronic hives represent a significant burden on global health, affecting individuals across all age groups, genders, and ethnicities. While acute urticaria is relatively common and often resolves within hours to weeks, chronic hives persist for longer durations, posing substantial challenges for patients and healthcare providers alike.

1. **Prevalence:** The prevalence of chronic hives varies widely across different populations and regions, with reported rates ranging from 0.1% to 1.0% in the general population. However, recent epidemiological data suggest that the prevalence of CIU may be higher than previously estimated, particularly in certain demographic groups and geographical areas.

2. **Incidence:** Studies investigating the annual incidence of chronic hives have reported rates ranging from 0.1% to 0.3%, indicating that a significant number of individuals develop the condition each year. The incidence of CIU appears to peak in early to middle adulthood, with a slight predilection for females compared to males.

Risk Factors:

Several factors may contribute to the development and exacerbation of chronic hives, including genetic predisposition, environmental triggers, comorbid conditions, and psychological factors.

1. **Genetic Factors:** Family history plays a significant role in

the development of chronic hives, with a higher prevalence observed among individuals with a family history of allergic diseases, including asthma, allergic rhinitis, and eczema. Twin studies have suggested a hereditary component to CIU, although specific genetic markers have yet to be identified conclusively.

2. **Environmental Triggers:** Exposure to certain environmental triggers, such as allergens, pollutants, and infectious agents, may precipitate or exacerbate chronic hives in susceptible individuals. Common allergens implicated in CIU include pollen, dust mites, animal dander, and certain foods, although the precise mechanisms underlying these associations remain incompletely understood.

3. **Comorbid Conditions:** Chronic hives frequently coexist with other allergic and autoimmune disorders, including asthma, allergic rhinitis, autoimmune thyroid diseases, and systemic lupus erythematosus (SLE). Additionally, conditions such as chronic infections (e.g., Helicobacter pylori), hormonal imbalances, and psychiatric disorders (e.g., anxiety, depression) may contribute to the pathogenesis of CIU and influence disease severity.

4. **Psychological Factors:** Psychological stress and emotional distress have been implicated as potential triggers or exacerbating factors in chronic hives. Patients with CIU often report higher levels of anxiety, depression, and perceived stress compared to the general population. Conversely, the presence of chronic hives can significantly impact patients' quality of life, leading to increased psychological morbidity and impaired social functioning.

Geographic and Demographic Variations:

The prevalence and incidence of chronic hives exhibit notable geographic and demographic variations, influenced by factors such as climate, socioeconomic status, access to healthcare, and cultural practices.

1. **Geographic Variations:** Studies have reported differences in the prevalence of chronic hives among various regions and countries, with higher rates observed in urban areas compared to rural settings. Environmental factors, including climate, pollution levels, and allergen exposure, may contribute to these geographic variations.

2. **Demographic Characteristics:** While chronic hives can affect individuals of all ages, genders, and ethnic backgrounds, certain demographic groups may be disproportionately affected. For example, females tend to have a higher prevalence of CIU compared to males, with some studies suggesting a female-to-male ratio of up to 2:1. Additionally, CIU appears to be more prevalent in adults than in children, although the condition can occur at any age.

Conclusion:

In conclusion, chronic hives represent a common and burdensome dermatological condition with significant implications for patients' quality of life and healthcare utilization. Epidemiological studies provide valuable insights into the prevalence, incidence, risk factors, and demographic characteristics associated with CIU, guiding efforts to improve diagnosis, treatment, and prevention strategies. By addressing the multifactorial nature of chronic hives and considering the diverse needs of affected individuals, healthcare professionals can better support patients in managing their symptoms and minimizing the impact of the condition on their daily lives.

Pathophysiology Overview of Chronic Hives

Chronic hives, also known as chronic idiopathic urticaria (CIU), is a complex dermatological disorder characterized by the recurrent appearance of wheals or hives on the skin, often accompanied by intense itching and discomfort. While the exact pathophysiology of CIU remains incompletely understood, significant advances have been made in elucidating the underlying mechanisms driving the development and persistence of this condition. A comprehensive understanding of the pathophysiology of chronic hives is essential for guiding therapeutic interventions and improving patient outcomes.

Mast Cell Activation:

Central to the pathogenesis of chronic hives is the dysregulated activation of mast cells, specialized immune cells found predominantly in the skin and mucosal tissues. Mast cells play a critical role in the body's immune response, releasing various inflammatory mediators, including histamine, leukotrienes, prostaglandins, and cytokines, upon activation. In chronic hives, mast cells become hypersensitive and hyperresponsive to a variety of stimuli, leading to excessive and uncontrolled release of these mediators into the surrounding tissue.

IgE-Mediated Mechanisms:

Traditionally associated with allergic reactions, IgE-mediated mechanisms have been implicated in a subset of chronic hives cases, particularly those with identifiable triggers such as food allergies or insect bites. In these instances, allergen-specific IgE antibodies bind to mast cell surface receptors, triggering mast cell degranulation and the release of histamine and other inflammatory mediators. However, the role of IgE in CIU is less clear, as many patients lack detectable allergen-specific IgE antibodies, suggesting the involvement of alternative pathways in mast cell activation.

Non-IgE Mediated Pathways:

In addition to IgE-mediated mechanisms, non-IgE pathways are thought to contribute to mast cell activation in chronic hives, particularly in cases where no specific trigger or allergen can be identified. These alternative pathways involve direct stimulation of mast cells by various factors, including physical stimuli (e.g., pressure, temperature changes), infectious agents (e.g., viral or bacterial antigens), autoantibodies, and neurogenic factors. The precise mechanisms by which these stimuli induce mast cell activation and degranulation are still under investigation but likely involve a combination of receptor-mediated signaling pathways and intracellular signaling cascades.

Autoimmune Mechanisms:

Growing evidence suggests that autoimmune mechanisms may play a significant role in a subset of chronic hives cases, particularly those characterized by autoantibodies targeting mast cell surface receptors or signaling molecules. These autoantibodies, which are detectable in the serum of some CIU patients, can trigger mast cell activation and degranulation, leading to the release of inflammatory mediators and the subsequent development of urticarial lesions. Autoimmune mechanisms may also involve the activation of complement pathways and the recruitment of immune cells to the site of inflammation, contributing to the chronicity and persistence of hives.

Neurogenic Factors:

Neurogenic factors, including the release of neuropeptides and neurotransmitters from sensory nerve fibers in the skin, are thought to modulate mast cell activity and contribute to the development of chronic hives. Stress, anxiety, and other emotional factors can activate the neuroendocrine system, leading to the release of neuropeptides such as substance P and calcitonin gene-related peptide (CGRP), which can directly stimulate mast cells and enhance their responsiveness to other stimuli. Additionally, the bidirectional communication between the nervous system and the immune system may perpetuate a cycle of chronic inflammation and hypersensitivity in CIU.

Conclusion:

In summary, chronic hives is a multifactorial disorder characterized by the dysregulated activation of mast cells and the release of inflammatory mediators in the skin. While the exact pathophysiology of CIU remains incompletely understood, current evidence suggests a complex interplay between immunological, neuroendocrine, and environmental factors in driving mast cell activation and the development of urticarial lesions. Further research is needed to elucidate the specific molecular mechanisms underlying chronic hives and to identify novel therapeutic targets for the treatment of this debilitating condition.

Clinical Presentation of Chronic Hives

Chronic hives, also known as chronic idiopathic urticaria (CIU), presents with a characteristic set of clinical features that distinguish it from other dermatological conditions. Understanding the clinical presentation of CIU is essential for accurate diagnosis, appropriate management, and effective patient care. This comprehensive overview will delve into the various aspects of the clinical presentation of chronic hives, including the appearance of lesions, associated symptoms, triggers, and complications.

Appearance of Lesions:

The hallmark feature of chronic hives is the presence of wheals or hives on the skin, which manifest as raised, erythematous (red), pruritic (itchy) plaques with well-defined borders. These wheals may vary in size, ranging from small papules to large patches, and can appear anywhere on the body, including the face, trunk, extremities, and mucous membranes. Individual lesions typically last for a few hours to a day before resolving spontaneously, although new lesions may continue to appear in different locations, resulting in a fluctuating and unpredictable course of the disease.

Associated Symptoms:

In addition to the characteristic wheals, patients with chronic hives may experience a range of associated symptoms, including pruritus (itching), erythema (redness), and, in some cases, angioedema. Pruritus is often the most distressing symptom for patients, leading to significant discomfort and impairment of daily activities. The intensity of itching can vary from mild to severe and may be exacerbated by factors such as heat, stress, and friction. Erythema accompanying the wheals results from the dilation of blood vessels in the skin and contributes to the characteristic red appearance of the lesions. Angioedema, characterized by deeper swelling in the dermis and subcutaneous tissues, may occur concurrently with or independently of wheals, typically affecting areas with loose connective tissue, such as the face, lips, eyelids, and genitalia. Angioedema can cause pain, discomfort, and functional impairment, particularly when it involves the upper airway, where it poses a risk of airway obstruction and respiratory compromise.

Triggers:

Identifying triggers that exacerbate or precipitate episodes of chronic hives is an essential aspect of managing the condition and preventing symptom recurrence. While many cases of CIU are considered idiopathic, meaning no specific trigger can be identified, certain factors have been implicated in exacerbating symptoms in susceptible individuals. Common triggers include physical stimuli such as pressure (dermatographism), cold, heat, sunlight (solar urticaria), vibration, and friction. Additionally, allergens such as foods, medications, insect stings, and environmental factors such as pollen, dust mites, and pet dander may trigger episodes of hives in some patients. Psychological stress and emotional factors have also been linked to exacerbations of chronic hives, although the precise mechanisms underlying these associations remain incompletely understood.

Complications:

While chronic hives is typically considered a benign and self-limited condition, certain complications may arise, particularly in severe or refractory cases. Persistent and recurrent itching can lead to excoriation (skin damage) and secondary bacterial infections, predisposing patients to complications such as cellulitis and folliculitis. Angioedema involving the upper airway can pose a risk of airway obstruction and respiratory compromise, necessitating prompt medical intervention. Furthermore, chronic hives can have a significant impact on patients' quality of life, leading to psychological distress, sleep disturbances, and impairment of daily activities. In severe cases, the physical and emotional burden of the disease may result in social isolation, depression, and decreased productivity.

Conclusion:

In conclusion, chronic hives is characterized by the recurrent appearance of wheals or hives on the skin, accompanied by itching, erythema, and, in some cases, angioedema. The clinical presentation of CIU is variable and may be influenced by factors such as triggers, comorbid conditions, and individual patient characteristics. Recognizing the characteristic features of chronic hives is essential for accurate diagnosis and appropriate management, which may include avoidance of triggers, pharmacological therapy, and patient education. By addressing the diverse needs of patients with chronic hives, healthcare providers can help improve symptom control, enhance quality of life, and minimize the impact of the disease on patients' overall well-being.

Diagnostic Criteria and Evaluation of Chronic Hives

Accurate diagnosis of chronic hives, also known as chronic idiopathic urticaria (CIU), is essential for guiding appropriate management strategies and improving patient outcomes. The diagnosis of CIU is primarily based on clinical evaluation, supported by a thorough medical history, physical examination, and, in some cases, additional diagnostic tests. This comprehensive overview will delve into the diagnostic criteria and evaluation methods used in the assessment of chronic hives, highlighting key considerations for healthcare providers.

Diagnostic Criteria:

The diagnosis of chronic hives is primarily clinical and is established based on the presence of recurrent wheals and/or angioedema lasting for at least six weeks, with no identifiable external cause or trigger. The diagnostic criteria for CIU include:

1. **Duration:** Symptoms of urticaria (wheals or angioedema) persisting for six weeks or longer.
2. **Recurrence:** Recurrent episodes of wheals and/or angioedema occurring intermittently over time.
3. **No Identifiable Cause:** Absence of a specific trigger or external factor identified through thorough history-taking and investigation.

It is important to differentiate CIU from acute urticaria, which typically resolves within six weeks and is often triggered by identifiable factors such as medications, infections, or allergic reactions. Chronic hives may present with a similar clinical appearance to acute urticaria; however, the duration of symptoms and lack of identifiable triggers distinguish CIU from its acute counterpart.

Clinical Evaluation:

The clinical evaluation of patients with suspected chronic hives begins with a detailed medical history and physical examination. Key components of the clinical assessment include:

1. **Medical History:** Healthcare providers should inquire about the onset, duration, frequency, and characteristics of the urticarial lesions, as well as any associated symptoms such as itching, swelling, and systemic manifestations. A comprehensive medical history should also include inquiries about potential triggers, previous treatments, underlying medical conditions, medication use, and family history of allergic diseases.

2. **Physical Examination:** A thorough physical examination is essential to assess the extent and distribution of urticarial lesions, as well as the presence of associated angioedema. Special attention should be given to areas commonly affected by hives, including the face, trunk, extremities, and mucous membranes. Signs of systemic involvement, such as fever, lymphadenopathy, or hepatosplenomegaly, should be evaluated to rule out underlying systemic diseases.

3. **Differential Diagnosis:** Differential diagnosis should be considered to exclude other dermatological conditions that may mimic the clinical presentation of chronic hives, such as urticarial vasculitis, eczema, contact dermatitis, erythema multiforme, and drug eruptions. Additional investigations may be warranted in cases where the diagnosis is uncertain or when alternative diagnoses are suspected.

Diagnostic Tests:

While the diagnosis of chronic hives is primarily clinical,

additional diagnostic tests may be indicated in certain situations to confirm the diagnosis, identify potential triggers, or assess for underlying systemic diseases. Diagnostic tests commonly used in the evaluation of chronic hives include:

1. **Laboratory Tests:** Laboratory investigations may include complete blood count (CBC), erythrocyte sedimentation rate (ESR), C-reactive protein (CRP), thyroid function tests (TFTs), autoimmune serology (e.g., antinuclear antibodies, rheumatoid factor), and serum IgE levels. These tests may help identify underlying systemic conditions or autoimmune disorders associated with chronic hives.

2. **Allergy Testing:** Allergy testing, including skin prick testing and specific IgE antibody assays, may be performed to identify potential allergens triggering urticarial reactions in some patients. However, it is important to recognize that allergy testing may be negative in many cases of chronic hives, particularly those classified as idiopathic.

3. **Provocation Tests:** Provocation tests, such as cold stimulation tests, pressure tests, and oral challenge tests with suspected food allergens or medications, may be conducted to induce urticarial reactions under controlled conditions. These tests can help identify physical triggers or specific allergens contributing to the development of chronic hives in some patients.

4. **Skin Biopsy:** In selected cases, a skin biopsy of urticarial lesions may be performed to rule out urticarial vasculitis or other histopathological features suggestive of alternative diagnoses. Skin biopsy findings in chronic hives typically reveal nonspecific changes, including perivascular inflammation, dermal edema, and mast cell degranulation.

Conclusion:

In conclusion, the diagnosis of chronic hives is established based on the presence of recurrent wheals and/or angioedema lasting for at least six weeks, with no identifiable external cause or trigger. Clinical evaluation, including a detailed medical history, physical examination, and, in some cases, additional diagnostic tests, is essential for accurate diagnosis and appropriate management of chronic hives. By employing a systematic approach to evaluation and considering the differential diagnosis, healthcare providers can effectively diagnose and manage patients with chronic hives, thereby improving symptom control and enhancing quality of life.

CHAPTER 2: IMMUNOLOGICAL BASIS OF CHRONIC HIVES

Role of Mast Cells in Urticaria

Mast cells, pivotal players in the immune system, are central to the pathogenesis of urticaria, a group of inflammatory skin disorders characterized by the sudden appearance of wheals or hives, angioedema, and intense itching. Understanding the intricate role of mast cells in urticaria is essential for unraveling the underlying mechanisms of the disease and developing targeted therapeutic strategies. This comprehensive overview will delve into the multifaceted role of mast cells in urticaria, encompassing their activation, degranulation, mediator release, and interactions with other immune cells.

Structure and Function of Mast Cells:

Mast cells are specialized immune cells derived from bone marrow precursors and distributed throughout the body, particularly in connective tissue, skin, mucosal surfaces, and blood vessels. Structurally, mast cells are characterized by granules containing a plethora of bioactive molecules, including histamine, proteases (such as tryptase and chymase), cytokines, chemokines, and growth factors. Upon activation, mast cells release these mediators into the surrounding tissue, triggering inflammatory responses and orchestrating immune reactions.

Activation of Mast Cells in Urticaria:

In urticaria, mast cells become hyperactivated in response to various stimuli, leading to their degranulation and the release of inflammatory mediators. While the exact triggers for mast cell activation in urticaria remain incompletely understood, several mechanisms have been implicated, including IgE-mediated pathways, non-IgE pathways, and neurogenic stimuli.

1. **IgE-Mediated Activation:** In allergic urticaria, antigen-specific IgE antibodies bind to high-affinity receptors (FcεRI) on mast cell surfaces, sensitizing the cells to subsequent exposure to allergens. Upon re-exposure to the allergen, cross-linking of IgE molecules on mast cells triggers intracellular signaling cascades, leading to mast cell degranulation and the release of preformed mediators such as histamine and tryptase.

2. **Non-IgE-Mediated Activation:** In non-allergic or idiopathic urticaria, mast cell activation can occur via non-IgE-mediated mechanisms, including direct stimulation by physical stimuli (e.g., pressure, temperature changes), infectious agents (e.g., viruses, bacteria), autoantibodies, and complement activation. These alternative pathways bypass the need for allergen-specific IgE antibodies and may contribute to the development of chronic urticaria in patients with no identifiable triggers.

3. **Neurogenic Activation:** Neurogenic stimuli, such as stress, anxiety, and emotional factors, can also activate mast cells via the release of neuropeptides and neurotransmitters from sensory nerve fibers in the

skin. Substance P, calcitonin gene-related peptide (CGRP), and vasoactive intestinal peptide (VIP) are among the neuropeptides implicated in mast cell activation and degranulation, promoting inflammation and pruritus in urticaria.

Mediator Release and Effects:

Following mast cell activation and degranulation, a cascade of inflammatory mediators is released into the surrounding tissue, triggering vasodilation, increased vascular permeability, smooth muscle contraction, and recruitment of immune cells. Histamine, the most well-known mediator released by mast cells, plays a central role in the pathogenesis of urticaria, causing vasodilation, edema formation, and pruritus. Other mediators released by mast cells, including leukotrienes, prostaglandins, cytokines, and chemokines, contribute to the inflammatory response and amplify the allergic cascade.

Interactions with Other Immune Cells:

Mast cells interact dynamically with other immune cells, including eosinophils, basophils, T cells, and dendritic cells, orchestrating complex immune responses in urticaria. Mast cell-derived mediators, such as histamine and cytokines, can recruit and activate eosinophils and basophils, amplifying the inflammatory response and contributing to tissue damage. Additionally, mast cells can modulate the function of T cells and dendritic cells, influencing adaptive immune responses and promoting the development of chronic inflammation in urticaria.

Therapeutic Implications:

Given the central role of mast cells in the pathogenesis of urticaria, therapeutic interventions targeting mast cell activation and mediator release represent promising approaches for the management of the disease. Antihistamines, the mainstay of treatment for urticaria, block the effects of histamine on target tissues and alleviate symptoms of itching and wheals. Additional therapies, including leukotriene receptor antagonists, corticosteroids, and immunomodulatory agents, target other mast cell-derived mediators and inflammatory pathways implicated in urticaria.

Conclusion:

In conclusion, mast cells play a pivotal role in the pathogenesis of urticaria, orchestrating inflammatory responses and immune reactions through the release of a diverse array of mediators. Understanding the complex interplay between mast cells, inflammatory mediators, and other immune cells is essential for elucidating the mechanisms underlying urticaria and developing targeted therapeutic strategies. By targeting mast cell activation and mediator release, healthcare providers can effectively manage symptoms and improve outcomes for patients with urticaria. Further research into the molecular mechanisms regulating mast cell function and interactions may uncover novel therapeutic targets for the treatment of this challenging dermatological condition.

IgE-mediated Mechanisms in Urticaria

IgE-mediated mechanisms represent a fundamental pathway in the pathogenesis of urticaria, a common inflammatory skin disorder characterized by the sudden appearance of wheals, angioedema, and intense itching. IgE, or immunoglobulin E, is an antibody class produced by the immune system in response to allergens and plays a central role in allergic reactions. In urticaria, IgE-mediated mechanisms contribute to mast cell activation and degranulation, leading to the release of inflammatory mediators and the development of characteristic urticarial lesions. This comprehensive overview will delve into the intricacies of IgE-mediated mechanisms in urticaria, encompassing the production of allergen-specific IgE antibodies, their binding to mast cell receptors, and the downstream signaling pathways that culminate in mast cell activation and mediator release.

Production of Allergen-specific IgE Antibodies:

The process of IgE-mediated sensitization begins when an individual is exposed to an allergen, such as pollen, animal dander, food proteins, or insect venom. In susceptible individuals, the allergen is recognized by antigen-presenting cells (APCs), such as dendritic cells or macrophages, and presented to naïve B lymphocytes. Upon activation, B cells undergo class switching and differentiation into plasma cells, which produce allergen-specific IgE antibodies.

These allergen-specific IgE antibodies have a high affinity for their cognate allergen and circulate in the bloodstream, binding to high-affinity IgE receptors (FcεRI) expressed on the surface of mast cells and basophils. Sensitization to specific allergens can occur following a single exposure or may require repeated exposures over time, depending on individual susceptibility and environmental factors.

Binding of IgE to Mast Cell Receptors:

The binding of allergen-specific IgE antibodies to FcεRI receptors on mast cells sensitizes the cells to subsequent exposure to the allergen. FcεRI receptors consist of four subunits: one IgE-binding α subunit, two signal-transducing β subunits, and one disulfide-linked γ subunit. Upon allergen binding, cross-linking of IgE molecules on adjacent FcεRI receptors occurs, leading to receptor clustering and the initiation of intracellular signaling cascades.

Downstream Signaling Pathways:

Cross-linking of IgE-bound FcεRI receptors initiates a series of signaling events within mast cells, ultimately resulting in mast cell activation and degranulation. The signaling pathways activated by FcεRI engagement include the phosphoinositide 3-kinase (PI3K)/Akt pathway, the mitogen-activated protein kinase (MAPK) pathway, and the calcium-dependent signaling pathway.

1. **PI3K/Akt Pathway:** Activation of PI3K leads to the generation of phosphatidylinositol (3,4,5)-trisphosphate (PIP3), which activates downstream effectors such as Akt. Akt activation promotes mast cell survival, proliferation, and cytokine production, contributing to the inflammatory response in urticaria.

2. **MAPK Pathway:** Activation of the MAPK pathway, including extracellular signal-regulated kinase (ERK), c-Jun N-terminal kinase (JNK), and p38 MAPK, leads to the phosphorylation of transcription factors such as activator protein-1 (AP-1) and nuclear factor-κB (NF-κB). These transcription factors regulate the expression of genes involved in inflammation, cytokine production, and mast cell activation.

3. **Calcium-dependent Signaling Pathway:** Cross-linking of IgE-bound FcεRI receptors induces calcium influx into mast cells, leading to the activation of calcium-dependent signaling pathways. Elevated intracellular calcium levels trigger the release of preformed mediators stored in mast cell granules, including histamine, tryptase, and cytokines.

Mast Cell Activation and Mediator Release:

The culmination of these signaling events is mast cell activation and degranulation, characterized by the rapid release of preformed mediators stored in mast cell granules. Histamine, the most well-known mast cell mediator, plays a central role in the pathogenesis of urticaria, causing vasodilation, increased vascular permeability, and itching. Tryptase, another protease released by mast cells, contributes to tissue inflammation and remodeling.

In addition to preformed mediators, mast cells also produce and release cytokines, chemokines, and lipid mediators in response to IgE-mediated activation. These soluble mediators amplify the inflammatory response, recruit immune cells to the site of inflammation, and modulate local immune responses, further exacerbating the symptoms of urticaria.

Therapeutic Implications:

Given the pivotal role of IgE-mediated mechanisms in urticaria, therapeutic interventions targeting IgE production, IgE receptor binding, or downstream signaling pathways represent promising strategies for the management of the disease. Antihistamines, the mainstay of treatment for urticaria, block the effects of histamine on target tissues and alleviate symptoms of itching and wheals. Additional therapies, including omalizumab (an anti-IgE monoclonal antibody) and small molecule inhibitors targeting intracellular signaling pathways, may provide relief for patients with refractory or severe urticaria.

Conclusion:

In conclusion, IgE-mediated mechanisms play a central role in the pathogenesis of urticaria, driving mast cell activation, mediator release, and the development of characteristic urticarial lesions. Understanding the intricate interplay between allergen-specific IgE antibodies, mast cell receptors, and downstream signaling pathways is essential for elucidating the mechanisms underlying urticaria and developing targeted therapeutic strategies. By targeting IgE-mediated mechanisms, healthcare providers can effectively manage symptoms and improve outcomes for patients with urticaria, enhancing their quality of life and reducing the burden of this debilitating skin disorder.

development of urticaria through neuroimmune interactions. Stress-induced release of neuropeptides and neurotransmitters, such as substance P, calcitonin gene-related peptide (CGRP), and vasoactive intestinal peptide (VIP), can directly activate mast cells and promote the release of inflammatory mediators. Additionally, stress-related alterations in neuroendocrine pathways, including the hypothalamic-pituitary-adrenal (HPA) axis and the autonomic nervous system, may influence mast cell function and exacerbate urticarial symptoms.

Therapeutic Implications:

Given the diverse array of triggers and mechanisms involved in non-IgE mediated pathways, therapeutic interventions targeting these pathways represent potential strategies for the management of urticaria. Identifying and avoiding specific triggers, such as physical stimuli or infectious agents, may help prevent symptom exacerbation in susceptible individuals. Additionally, pharmacological therapies targeting mast cell activation and mediator release, including antihistamines, leukotriene receptor antagonists, and mast cell stabilizers, may provide symptomatic relief for patients with urticaria.

Conclusion:

In conclusion, non-IgE mediated pathways play a significant role in the pathogenesis of urticaria, contributing to mast cell activation and the release of inflammatory mediators through physical stimuli, infectious agents, autoantibodies, complement activation, and neurogenic factors. Understanding the diverse array of triggers and mechanisms involved in non-IgE mediated pathways is essential for comprehensively addressing the heterogeneity of urticaria and developing targeted therapeutic interventions. By targeting non-IgE mediated pathways, healthcare providers can effectively manage symptoms and improve outcomes for patients with urticaria, reducing the burden of this chronic inflammatory skin disorder.

Autoimmune Mechanisms in Chronic Hives

Chronic hives, also known as chronic idiopathic urticaria (CIU), is a complex dermatological disorder characterized by the recurrent appearance of wheals or hives on the skin, often accompanied by intense itching and discomfort. While the exact etiology of CIU remains elusive in many cases, accumulating evidence suggests that autoimmune mechanisms play a significant role in the pathogenesis of the disease. Autoimmune mechanisms in CIU involve the production of autoantibodies targeting mast cell surface receptors or signaling molecules, leading to mast cell activation and the release of inflammatory mediators. This comprehensive overview will delve into the intricate interplay between autoimmunity and chronic hives, encompassing the production of autoantibodies, mast cell activation, and therapeutic implications.

Production of Autoantibodies:

Autoimmune mechanisms in CIU are characterized by the production of autoantibodies targeting mast cell surface receptors or IgE molecules, leading to mast cell activation and the release of inflammatory mediators. Autoantibodies against IgE receptors (FcεRI or FcεRII/CD23) or IgE molecules can cross-link mast cell receptors, initiating intracellular signaling cascades and promoting mast cell degranulation. Additionally, autoantibodies targeting other mast cell surface antigens, such as IgG antibodies against the high-affinity IgE receptor (FcεRI), have been implicated in the pathogenesis of CIU.

Mast Cell Activation:

Upon binding of autoantibodies to mast cell surface receptors, cross-linking of receptor molecules occurs, leading to the activation of intracellular signaling pathways and the release of inflammatory mediators. Mast cell activation in CIU results in the rapid release of preformed mediators stored in mast cell granules, including histamine, tryptase, and cytokines. These mediators contribute to the development of wheals, angioedema, and pruritus characteristic of CIU.

Autoimmune Subtypes of CIU:

Autoimmune mechanisms in CIU encompass a spectrum of subtypes, including chronic spontaneous urticaria (CSU) and autoimmune urticaria. CSU is characterized by the recurrent appearance of wheals or hives without an identifiable external trigger, while autoimmune urticaria is distinguished by the presence of autoantibodies targeting mast cell surface receptors or IgE molecules. Autoimmune urticaria may present with distinct clinical features, including refractoriness to standard therapies and a more severe and persistent disease course.

Role of Autoantibodies in Pathogenesis:

Autoantibodies in CIU can directly activate mast cells and basophils, leading to the release of inflammatory mediators and the development of urticarial lesions. Additionally, autoantibodies may modulate mast cell function indirectly by enhancing the effects of IgE-mediated mast cell activation or promoting complement activation. Autoantibodies against IgE receptors or IgE molecules may cross-link mast cell receptors, amplifying intracellular signaling cascades and exacerbating mast cell degranulation.

Diagnostic Implications:

The presence of autoantibodies targeting mast cell surface receptors or IgE molecules may have diagnostic implications in CIU, particularly in cases refractory to standard therapies. Detection of autoantibodies in serum samples using immunoassays, such as enzyme-linked immunosorbent assays

(ELISA) or immunoblotting techniques, may aid in the diagnosis and classification of autoimmune subtypes of CIU. However, the clinical significance of autoantibodies in CIU remains a subject of ongoing research, and further studies are needed to elucidate their role in disease pathogenesis and therapeutic response.

Therapeutic Implications:

Therapeutic strategies targeting autoimmune mechanisms in CIU aim to suppress mast cell activation and inflammatory mediator release, thereby alleviating symptoms and improving disease control. Omalizumab, a monoclonal antibody targeting IgE, has shown efficacy in the treatment of refractory CIU, particularly in patients with evidence of autoantibodies targeting IgE receptors. Additionally, immunomodulatory agents such as cyclosporine and intravenous immunoglobulin (IVIG) may be considered in severe or refractory cases of CIU with autoimmune features.

Conclusion:

In conclusion, autoimmune mechanisms play a significant role in the pathogenesis of chronic hives, contributing to mast cell activation and the release of inflammatory mediators through the production of autoantibodies targeting mast cell surface receptors or IgE molecules. Autoimmune subtypes of CIU, including chronic spontaneous urticaria (CSU) and autoimmune urticaria, may present with distinct clinical features and therapeutic challenges. Understanding the intricate interplay between autoimmunity and chronic hives is essential for guiding diagnostic evaluation and therapeutic decision-making in patients with refractory or autoimmune subtypes of CIU. Further research into the mechanisms underlying autoimmune mechanisms in CIU may uncover novel therapeutic targets and improve outcomes for patients with this debilitating dermatological condition.

Neurogenic Factors in Urticaria

Urticaria, characterized by the sudden onset of wheals or hives on the skin, often accompanied by intense itching and discomfort, is a multifaceted dermatological condition with various underlying mechanisms. While immune-mediated pathways, including IgE-mediated and autoimmune mechanisms, have been extensively studied in urticaria, emerging evidence suggests a significant role for neurogenic factors in the pathogenesis of the disease. Neurogenic factors encompass a wide range of stimuli and pathways originating from the nervous system, including stress, anxiety, neurotransmitters, and neuropeptides, which can modulate mast cell activity and contribute to the development and exacerbation of urticarial symptoms. This comprehensive overview will explore the intricate interplay between neurogenic factors and urticaria, encompassing the effects of stress, neurotransmitters, neuropeptides, and therapeutic implications.

Effects of Stress and Anxiety:

Stress and anxiety are known triggers for urticaria, with many patients reporting exacerbation of symptoms during periods of emotional distress or psychological upheaval. The connection between stress and urticaria is mediated through neuroendocrine pathways, including the hypothalamic-pituitary-adrenal (HPA) axis and the autonomic nervous system. Stress-induced activation of the HPA axis leads to the release of cortisol, a stress hormone that can modulate immune responses and mast cell activity. Additionally, sympathetic nervous system activation during stress can stimulate mast cell degranulation through the release of neurotransmitters such as norepinephrine.

Neurotransmitters:

Neurotransmitters released by the nervous system play a crucial role in modulating mast cell activity and immune responses in urticaria. Norepinephrine, a key neurotransmitter released by sympathetic nerve fibers, can directly activate mast cells and enhance histamine release, leading to the development of wheals and pruritus. Conversely, acetylcholine, released by parasympathetic nerve fibers, may exert inhibitory effects on mast cell degranulation, providing a counter-regulatory mechanism in the nervous system.

Neuropeptides:

Neuropeptides, such as substance P, calcitonin gene-related peptide (CGRP), and vasoactive intestinal peptide (VIP), are released from sensory nerve fibers in the skin and can modulate mast cell activity and immune responses in urticaria. Substance P, a neuropeptide associated with pain transmission and neurogenic inflammation, can directly activate mast cells and promote the release of inflammatory mediators, including histamine and cytokines. CGRP, another neuropeptide involved in vasodilation and nociception, may enhance mast cell degranulation and contribute to the development of urticarial lesions. VIP, a potent vasodilator and anti-inflammatory peptide, may exert inhibitory effects on mast cell activation and inflammatory responses, providing a protective role in the skin.

Pathophysiological Mechanisms:

Neurogenic factors in urticaria exert their effects through a variety of pathophysiological mechanisms, including direct stimulation of mast cells, modulation of immune responses, and alteration of vascular permeability. Stress-induced activation of the HPA axis and sympathetic nervous system can lead to the release of cortisol and norepinephrine, respectively, which can directly activate mast cells and enhance histamine release. Additionally, neuropeptides such as substance P and CGRP can promote mast cell degranulation and inflammatory mediator release, contributing to the development of urticarial lesions.

Therapeutic Implications:

Therapeutic strategies targeting neurogenic factors in urticaria aim to modulate mast cell activity and alleviate symptoms by reducing stress, blocking neurotransmitter receptors, or interfering with neuropeptide signaling pathways. Stress management techniques, such as relaxation exercises, mindfulness-based stress reduction, and cognitive-behavioral therapy, may help reduce symptom severity and improve quality of life in patients with stress-induced urticaria. Pharmacological interventions targeting neurotransmitter receptors, such as beta-blockers or alpha-2 adrenergic agonists, may provide symptomatic relief by blocking sympathetic nervous system activation and reducing mast cell degranulation. Additionally, inhibitors of neuropeptide receptors, such as neurokinin-1 receptor antagonists or CGRP receptor antagonists, may offer therapeutic potential in the management of neurogenic urticaria.

Conclusion:

In conclusion, neurogenic factors play a significant role in the pathogenesis of urticaria, contributing to mast cell activation, inflammatory mediator release, and the development of urticarial lesions. Stress, anxiety, neurotransmitters, and neuropeptides originating from the nervous system can modulate mast cell activity and immune responses in urticaria, influencing disease severity and symptomatology. Understanding the intricate interplay between neurogenic factors and urticaria is essential for guiding therapeutic interventions and improving outcomes for patients with this debilitating dermatological condition. Further research into the mechanisms underlying neurogenic urticaria may uncover novel therapeutic targets and therapeutic strategies, paving the way for more effective management of this challenging disease.

CHAPTER 3: MOLECULAR MECHANISMS AND BIOCHEMISTRY OF CHRONIC HIVES

Histamine Release and Metabolism in Urticaria

Histamine, a biogenic amine synthesized from the amino acid histidine, plays a central role in the pathogenesis of urticaria, a common inflammatory skin disorder characterized by the sudden appearance of wheals, angioedema, and intense itching. Histamine release and metabolism are tightly regulated processes that involve the synthesis, storage, release, and degradation of histamine by various cells and enzymes within the body. Understanding the intricate dynamics of histamine release and metabolism is essential for elucidating the mechanisms underlying urticaria and developing targeted therapeutic strategies. This comprehensive overview will delve into the multifaceted aspects of histamine release and metabolism in urticaria, encompassing histamine synthesis, storage, release mechanisms, receptor interactions, and degradation pathways.

Histamine Synthesis:

Histamine synthesis occurs primarily in mast cells, basophils, and enterochromaffin-like cells in the gastrointestinal tract. The enzymatic conversion of histidine to histamine is catalyzed by the enzyme histidine decarboxylase, which is expressed predominantly in mast cells and basophils. Histamine synthesis is regulated by various factors, including intracellular calcium levels, cytokines, and growth factors, which modulate the expression and activity of histidine decarboxylase in response to physiological and pathological stimuli.

Histamine Storage:

Once synthesized, histamine is stored in cytoplasmic granules within mast cells and basophils, where it remains in an inactive form until released in response to appropriate stimuli. Histamine storage within mast cell granules is facilitated by vesicular monoamine transporter-2 (VMAT-2), a transmembrane protein that transports histamine from the cytoplasm into secretory vesicles for storage. Mast cells contain large quantities of histamine, with each mast cell capable of storing and releasing significant amounts of histamine upon activation.

Histamine Release Mechanisms:

Histamine release from mast cells and basophils can occur through various mechanisms, including immunological, non-immunological, and neurogenic pathways. Immunological histamine release occurs in response to cross-linking of IgE antibodies bound to high-affinity IgE receptors (FcεRI) on mast cell surfaces, triggered by exposure to allergens or immune complexes. Non-immunological histamine release can be induced by physical stimuli, such as pressure, temperature changes, or drugs, which directly activate mast cells and trigger degranulation. Neurogenic histamine release involves the stimulation of sensory nerve fibers in the skin by neuropeptides, neurotransmitters, or stress hormones, leading to mast cell activation and histamine release.

Histamine Receptors and Effects:

Histamine exerts its biological effects by binding to specific receptors expressed on target cells, including four distinct receptor subtypes: H1, H2, H3, and H4 receptors. H1 receptors are primarily expressed on vascular endothelial cells, smooth muscle cells, and sensory nerve fibers in the skin, where they mediate vasodilation, increased vascular permeability, and pruritus. H2 receptors are predominantly found on gastric parietal cells, where they stimulate gastric acid secretion and regulate immune responses. H3 receptors are primarily located in the central nervous system, where they modulate neurotransmitter release and synaptic transmission. H4 receptors are expressed on various immune cells, including mast cells, basophils, and T cells, where they regulate immune cell activation and chemotaxis.

Histamine Degradation Pathways:

Histamine degradation occurs through two main pathways: enzymatic degradation by histamine N-methyltransferase (HNMT) and diamine oxidase (DAO), and non-enzymatic degradation by histamine oxidase. HNMT is predominantly expressed in the central nervous system and liver, where it catalyzes the methylation of histamine to form N-methylhistamine, a less active metabolite. DAO, also known as histaminase, is primarily found in the gastrointestinal tract, where it catalyzes the oxidative deamination of histamine to form imidazole acetaldehyde, which is further metabolized to imidazole acetic acid. Histamine oxidase, present in various tissues, including skin and liver, can oxidize histamine to form inactive metabolites, such as imidazole acetaldehyde and imidazole acetic acid.

Role of Histamine in Urticaria:

Histamine is a key mediator of inflammation and pruritus in urticaria, exerting its effects through H1 receptors on target cells in the skin and other tissues. Upon release from activated mast cells and basophils, histamine binds to H1 receptors on vascular endothelial cells, leading to vasodilation and increased vascular permeability, which contribute to the formation of wheals and angioedema. Additionally, histamine binding to H1 receptors on sensory nerve fibers in the skin induces itching and pruritus, which are characteristic symptoms of urticaria.

Therapeutic Implications:

Therapeutic strategies targeting histamine release and metabolism in urticaria aim to block histamine effects, reduce mast cell activation, and enhance histamine degradation. Antihistamines, the mainstay of treatment for urticaria, competitively antagonize H1 receptors, thereby blocking the effects of histamine on target tissues and alleviating symptoms of itching and wheals. Additionally, inhibitors of histamine synthesis or mast cell degranulation, such as corticosteroids, leukotriene receptor antagonists, and mast cell stabilizers, may provide symptomatic relief by reducing histamine release and inflammatory responses. Enhancing histamine degradation through supplementation with DAO or histamine-reducing diets may also offer therapeutic potential in the management of histamine intolerance and urticaria.

Conclusion:

In conclusion, histamine release and metabolism play a central role in the pathogenesis of urticaria, contributing to the development of wheals, angioedema, and pruritus characteristic of the disease. Understanding the intricate dynamics of histamine synthesis, storage, release mechanisms, receptor interactions, and degradation pathways is essential for elucidating the mechanisms underlying urticaria and developing targeted therapeutic strategies. By targeting histamine release and metabolism, healthcare providers can effectively manage symptoms and improve outcomes for patients with urticaria, enhancing their quality of life and reducing the burden of this chronic inflammatory skin disorder. Further research into novel therapeutic targets and interventions may offer new insights into the treatment of urticaria and improve patient care in the future.

Pro-inflammatory Cytokines in Urticaria

Urticaria, a common dermatological condition characterized by the sudden onset of wheals, angioedema, and pruritus, is driven by a complex interplay of inflammatory mediators, including pro-inflammatory cytokines. Cytokines are small proteins secreted by various cells of the immune system, such as mast cells, T cells, and macrophages, that regulate immune responses and inflammation. In urticaria, pro-inflammatory cytokines play a pivotal role in orchestrating the inflammatory cascade, promoting mast cell activation, vascular permeability, and leukocyte recruitment, ultimately leading to the development of urticarial lesions. This comprehensive overview will delve into the multifaceted role of pro-inflammatory cytokines in urticaria, encompassing their synthesis, release, signaling pathways, and therapeutic implications.

Synthesis and Release of Pro-inflammatory Cytokines:

Pro-inflammatory cytokines implicated in urticaria, including interleukin-1 (IL-1), interleukin-6 (IL-6), interleukin-8 (IL-8), and tumor necrosis factor-alpha (TNF-α), are synthesized and released by various immune cells in response to inflammatory stimuli. Mast cells, the primary effector cells in urticaria, are capable of producing and secreting a wide range of pro-inflammatory cytokines upon activation, including TNF-α, IL-1, and IL-6, which amplify the inflammatory response and contribute to the pathogenesis of urticaria. Additionally, infiltrating immune cells, such as T cells and macrophages, may release pro-inflammatory cytokines in the lesional skin, further exacerbating inflammation and tissue damage.

Role of Pro-inflammatory Cytokines in Mast Cell Activation:

Pro-inflammatory cytokines play a critical role in mast cell activation and degranulation in urticaria, amplifying the effects of IgE-mediated and non-IgE mediated stimuli. TNF-α, IL-1, and IL-6 can directly activate mast cells and enhance their responsiveness to IgE cross-linking, leading to increased histamine release and inflammatory mediator production. Additionally, pro-inflammatory cytokines may induce the expression of adhesion molecules and chemokines on endothelial cells, facilitating the recruitment of inflammatory cells to the site of inflammation and promoting tissue infiltration and damage.

Effects of Pro-inflammatory Cytokines on Vascular Permeability:

Pro-inflammatory cytokines exert potent effects on vascular endothelial cells, increasing vascular permeability and facilitating the extravasation of plasma proteins and immune cells into the surrounding tissues. IL-1 and TNF-α can directly stimulate endothelial cells to express adhesion molecules such as intercellular adhesion molecule-1 (ICAM-1) and vascular cell adhesion molecule-1 (VCAM-1), which promote leukocyte-endothelial cell interactions and leukocyte transmigration. IL-8, a potent chemokine released by mast cells and macrophages, further enhances vascular permeability and leukocyte recruitment by inducing endothelial cell activation and chemotaxis.

Inflammatory Signaling Pathways:

Pro-inflammatory cytokines exert their effects through the activation of intracellular signaling pathways, including the nuclear factor-kappa B (NF-κB) pathway, the mitogen-activated protein kinase (MAPK) pathway, and the Janus kinase/signal transducer and activator of transcription (JAK/STAT) pathway. Upon binding to their respective receptors on target cells, pro-inflammatory cytokines initiate signaling cascades that culminate in the activation of transcription factors, such as NF-κB and STATs, which regulate the expression of genes involved in inflammation, immune responses, and cell survival. Dysregulation of these signaling pathways may contribute to chronic inflammation and tissue damage in urticaria.

Therapeutic Implications:

Therapeutic strategies targeting pro-inflammatory cytokines in urticaria aim to suppress inflammation, reduce mast cell activation, and alleviate symptoms by blocking cytokine production or signaling pathways. Biologic agents, such as monoclonal antibodies targeting TNF-α (e.g., infliximab) or IL-1 (e.g., anakinra), have shown efficacy in the treatment of refractory urticaria, particularly in patients with evidence of elevated cytokine levels or inflammatory skin lesions. Additionally, small molecule inhibitors targeting intracellular signaling pathways, such as NF-κB inhibitors or JAK inhibitors, may offer therapeutic potential in the management of chronic urticaria with pro-inflammatory cytokine involvement.

Conclusion:

In conclusion, pro-inflammatory cytokines play a pivotal role in the pathogenesis of urticaria, driving mast cell activation, vascular permeability, and leukocyte recruitment through a complex network of signaling pathways. Understanding the multifaceted role of pro-inflammatory cytokines in urticaria is essential for elucidating the mechanisms underlying inflammation and tissue damage and developing targeted therapeutic interventions. By targeting pro-inflammatory cytokines and their signaling pathways, healthcare providers can effectively manage inflammation and improve outcomes for patients with urticaria, reducing the burden of this chronic inflammatory skin disorder. Further research into the role of pro-inflammatory cytokines in urticaria may uncover novel therapeutic targets and strategies, paving the way for more personalized and effective treatments in the future.

Immunoglobulin Pathways in Urticaria

Urticaria, a common dermatological condition characterized by the sudden appearance of wheals, angioedema, and pruritus, involves a complex interplay of immune mechanisms, including immunoglobulin pathways. Immunoglobulins, also known as antibodies, are key components of the adaptive immune system that recognize and bind to specific antigens, triggering immune responses against pathogens and foreign substances. In urticaria, immunoglobulin pathways encompass various mechanisms involving IgE-mediated hypersensitivity reactions, autoantibodies targeting mast cell surface receptors, and immune complex deposition, which contribute to mast cell activation, inflammation, and tissue damage. This comprehensive overview will delve into the multifaceted role of immunoglobulin pathways in urticaria, encompassing IgE-mediated mechanisms, autoimmune pathways, and immune complex deposition.

IgE-Mediated Mechanisms:

IgE-mediated mechanisms represent a major pathway in the pathogenesis of urticaria, particularly in allergic and atopic individuals. Upon exposure to allergens, such as food proteins, pollen, or insect venom, antigen-specific IgE antibodies are produced by plasma cells and bind to high-affinity IgE receptors (FcɛRI) on the surface of mast cells and basophils. Subsequent exposure to the same allergen cross-links IgE receptors on mast cells, triggering intracellular signaling cascades that lead to mast cell degranulation and the release of inflammatory mediators, including histamine, leukotrienes, and cytokines. This IgE-mediated mast cell activation results in the characteristic wheals, angioedema, and pruritus seen in urticaria.

Autoimmune Pathways:

Autoimmune mechanisms play a significant role in a subset of patients with chronic urticaria, particularly those with autoimmune urticaria subtypes such as chronic spontaneous urticaria (CSU) and autoimmune urticaria. In these cases, autoantibodies targeting mast cell surface receptors or IgE antibodies may lead to mast cell activation and the release of inflammatory mediators. Autoantibodies against IgE receptors (FcεRI or FcεRII/CD23), IgE molecules, or other mast cell surface antigens can cross-link mast cell receptors, initiating intracellular signaling cascades and promoting mast cell degranulation. Additionally, complement activation and immune complex deposition may contribute to tissue inflammation and vascular permeability in autoimmune urticaria.

Immune Complex Deposition:

Immune complex deposition represents another immunoglobulin pathway implicated in the pathogenesis of urticaria, particularly in urticarial vasculitis and serum sickness-like reactions. Immune complexes, consisting of antigen-antibody complexes, can deposit in small blood vessels within the skin and other tissues, leading to complement activation, leukocyte recruitment, and tissue damage. In urticarial vasculitis, immune complex-mediated inflammation results in the characteristic wheals and vascular lesions seen in urticarial vasculitis, accompanied by systemic symptoms such as fever and arthralgia. Similarly, serum sickness-like reactions, triggered by exposure to medications or foreign proteins, may present with urticarial lesions and systemic symptoms due to immune complex deposition and complement activation.

Diagnostic Implications:

The presence of immunoglobulin-mediated mechanisms in urticaria may have diagnostic implications, particularly in cases refractory to standard therapies or with atypical clinical features. Detection of allergen-specific IgE antibodies in serum samples using immunoassays, such as enzyme-linked immunosorbent assays (ELISA) or skin prick testing, may aid in identifying IgE-mediated triggers in allergic urticaria. Additionally, measurement of autoantibodies targeting mast cell surface receptors or IgE molecules may help classify autoimmune subtypes of urticaria and guide therapeutic decision-making. Evaluation of complement levels and immune complex deposition may be indicated in patients with suspected urticarial vasculitis or serum sickness-like reactions, particularly in those with systemic symptoms or cutaneous vasculitis.

Therapeutic Implications:

Therapeutic strategies targeting immunoglobulin pathways in urticaria aim to suppress immune responses, reduce mast cell activation, and alleviate symptoms by blocking antibody production or inhibiting immune complex formation. Antihistamines, the mainstay of treatment for urticaria, competitively antagonize histamine effects and may indirectly suppress IgE-mediated mast cell activation. Additionally, immunomodulatory agents such as corticosteroids, immunosuppressants, and biologic therapies may be considered in refractory cases of urticaria with autoimmune features or immune complex-mediated inflammation. Desensitization therapy, aimed at inducing tolerance to specific allergens, may be beneficial in allergic urticaria by reducing allergen-specific IgE production and mast cell sensitization.

Conclusion:

In conclusion, immunoglobulin pathways play a significant

role in the pathogenesis of urticaria, encompassing IgE-mediated mechanisms, autoimmune pathways, and immune complex deposition. Understanding the multifaceted role of immunoglobulin pathways in urticaria is essential for elucidating the mechanisms underlying inflammation and tissue damage and developing targeted therapeutic interventions. By targeting immunoglobulin pathways, healthcare providers can effectively manage inflammation and improve outcomes for patients with urticaria, reducing the burden of this chronic inflammatory skin disorder. Further research into the role of immunoglobulin pathways in urticaria may uncover novel therapeutic targets and strategies, paving the way for more personalized and effective treatments in the future.

Complement Activation in Urticaria

Urticaria, a dermatological condition characterized by the sudden appearance of wheals, angioedema, and pruritus, involves a complex interplay of immune mechanisms, including complement activation. The complement system, a key component of the innate immune system, consists of a cascade of proteins that interact to opsonize pathogens, stimulate inflammation, and lyse target cells. In urticaria, dysregulation of the complement system can lead to excessive complement activation, resulting in tissue inflammation, vascular permeability, and mast cell activation. This comprehensive overview will delve into the multifaceted role of complement activation in urticaria, encompassing its pathways, regulation, involvement in urticarial subtypes, and therapeutic implications.

Complement Pathways:

The complement system comprises three main activation pathways: the classical pathway, the lectin pathway, and the alternative pathway. The classical pathway is initiated by the binding of C1q to antigen-antibody complexes, leading to the activation of downstream complement components, including C4 and C2, and the formation of the C3 convertase. The lectin pathway is activated by the binding of mannose-binding lectin (MBL) or ficolins to microbial carbohydrates, leading to the activation of MBL-associated serine proteases (MASPs) and subsequent cleavage of C4 and C2. The alternative pathway is constitutively active at low levels and can be spontaneously activated by hydrolysis of C3, leading to the formation of the alternative pathway C3 convertase (C3bBb).

Regulation of Complement Activation:

Complement activation is tightly regulated by various soluble and membrane-bound regulators to prevent excessive tissue damage and inflammation. Soluble regulators, such as factor H and factor I, inhibit the formation and stabilize the decay of C3 convertases, thereby limiting complement amplification. Membrane-bound regulators, including decay-accelerating factor (DAF) and membrane cofactor protein (MCP), accelerate the decay of C3 convertases and promote the degradation of C3b, preventing complement deposition on host cells. Dysregulation of complement regulation can result in excessive complement activation and tissue injury, as seen in complement-mediated diseases such as urticaria.

Role of Complement Activation in Urticarial Subtypes:

Complement activation has been implicated in various subtypes of urticaria, including urticarial vasculitis, autoimmune urticaria, and drug-induced urticaria. In urticarial vasculitis, immune complex deposition triggers complement activation, leading to inflammation and vascular damage in small blood vessels within the skin. Complement-mediated inflammation contributes to the characteristic wheals and vascular lesions seen in urticarial vasculitis, accompanied by systemic symptoms such as fever and arthralgia. Similarly, in autoimmune urticaria, autoantibodies targeting mast cell surface receptors or IgE molecules can activate complement, leading to mast cell degranulation and the release of inflammatory mediators. Drug-induced urticaria may also involve complement activation, either directly through drug-induced complement activation or indirectly through immune complex formation.

Complement Activation and Mast Cell Activation:

Complement activation products, including C3a and C5a, are potent anaphylatoxins that can directly activate mast cells and promote the release of histamine and other inflammatory mediators. C3a and C5a bind to their respective receptors on mast cells, triggering intracellular signaling cascades that lead to mast cell degranulation and the release of preformed mediators stored in mast cell granules. Additionally, complement activation products can enhance IgE-mediated mast cell activation by synergizing with IgE-dependent stimuli, amplifying inflammatory responses and exacerbating urticarial symptoms.

Therapeutic Implications:

Therapeutic strategies targeting complement activation in urticaria aim to suppress complement activation, reduce inflammation, and alleviate symptoms by blocking complement components or inhibiting complement activation pathways. In urticarial vasculitis, immunosuppressive agents such as corticosteroids or rituximab may be used to suppress immune complex formation and complement activation. In autoimmune urticaria, monoclonal antibodies targeting complement components or complement inhibitors, such as eculizumab or C1 esterase inhibitor, may be considered in refractory cases with evidence of complement-mediated inflammation. Additionally, antihistamines and other symptomatic treatments may provide relief by attenuating mast cell activation and histamine release downstream of complement activation.

Conclusion:

In conclusion, complement activation plays a significant role in the pathogenesis of urticaria, contributing to tissue inflammation, mast cell activation, and urticarial lesions. Understanding the multifaceted role of complement activation in urticaria is essential for elucidating the mechanisms underlying inflammation and tissue damage and developing targeted therapeutic interventions. By targeting complement activation pathways, healthcare providers can effectively manage inflammation and improve outcomes for patients with urticaria, reducing the burden of this chronic inflammatory skin disorder. Further research into the role of complement activation in urticaria may uncover novel therapeutic targets and strategies, paving the way for more personalized and effective treatments in the future.

Cellular Signaling Pathways in Urticaria

Urticaria, characterized by the sudden onset of wheals, angioedema, and pruritus, is a complex dermatological condition involving dysregulation of cellular signaling pathways. Cellular signaling pathways orchestrate various cellular responses, including inflammation, immune activation, and tissue remodeling, all of which contribute to the pathogenesis of urticaria. Understanding the intricate interplay of cellular signaling pathways in urticaria is essential for elucidating the mechanisms underlying disease development and identifying potential therapeutic targets. This comprehensive overview will delve into the multifaceted role of cellular signaling pathways in urticaria, encompassing key signaling cascades, their regulation, and their implications for disease management.

Key Signaling Cascades:

Several signaling pathways play critical roles in the pathogenesis of urticaria, including the nuclear factor-kappa B (NF-κB) pathway, the mitogen-activated protein kinase (MAPK) pathway, and the phosphoinositide 3-kinase (PI3K)/ Akt pathway. Activation of these signaling cascades occurs in response to various stimuli, including allergens, cytokines, and neurotransmitters, leading to the expression of pro-inflammatory genes, cytokine production, and cell activation. Dysregulation of these signaling pathways can lead to excessive inflammation, tissue damage, and the development of urticarial lesions.

NF-κB Pathway:

The NF-κB pathway plays a central role in regulating inflammatory responses and immune activation in urticaria. Activation of NF-κB occurs in response to pro-inflammatory cytokines, such as tumor necrosis factor-alpha (TNF-α) and interleukin-1 (IL-1), or allergen exposure, leading to the nuclear translocation of NF-κB transcription factors and the induction of target gene expression. NF-κB target genes include cytokines, chemokines, adhesion molecules, and inflammatory mediators, which promote inflammation, leukocyte recruitment, and tissue damage in urticaria.

MAPK Pathway:

The MAPK pathway is another key signaling cascade involved in urticaria pathogenesis, regulating cell proliferation, differentiation, and inflammation. The MAPK pathway consists of three main branches: the extracellular signal-regulated kinase (ERK), c-Jun N-terminal kinase (JNK), and p38 MAPK pathways. Activation of MAPKs occurs in response to growth factors, cytokines, and environmental stressors, leading to the phosphorylation of downstream transcription factors and the induction of target gene expression. MAPK-mediated signaling promotes mast cell activation, cytokine production, and leukocyte recruitment in urticaria, contributing to the development of urticarial lesions.

PI3K/Akt Pathway:

The PI3K/Akt pathway plays a critical role in cell survival, proliferation, and migration in urticaria. Activation of PI3K leads to the generation of phosphatidylinositol 3,4,5-triphosphate (PIP3), which recruits and activates Akt at the plasma membrane. Akt activation promotes cell survival and proliferation by phosphorylating downstream targets involved in cell cycle progression and apoptosis regulation. Dysregulation of the PI3K/Akt pathway has been implicated in the pathogenesis of urticaria, contributing to mast cell survival, cytokine production, and inflammatory responses.

Regulation of Signaling Pathways:

Cellular signaling pathways in urticaria are tightly regulated by various mechanisms to maintain homeostasis and prevent excessive inflammation. Negative regulators, such as phosphatases and ubiquitin ligases, counteract signaling pathway activation by dephosphorylating or degrading signaling molecules, terminating signaling cascades and attenuating cellular responses. Additionally, feedback loops and cross-talk between signaling pathways provide further regulation and coordination of cellular responses in urticaria. Dysregulation of signaling pathway regulators can lead to aberrant signaling pathway activation and contribute to disease pathogenesis.

Implications for Disease Management:

Understanding the role of cellular signaling pathways in urticaria has important implications for disease management and therapeutic intervention. Targeting key signaling molecules or pathways involved in urticaria pathogenesis may provide novel therapeutic approaches for the treatment of this condition. Small molecule inhibitors targeting signaling pathway components, such as MAPK inhibitors or PI3K/Akt inhibitors, may offer therapeutic potential in the management of refractory urticaria by suppressing inflammation and reducing mast cell activation. Additionally, biologic agents targeting cytokines or cytokine receptors involved in signaling pathway activation, such as TNF-α inhibitors or IL-1 receptor antagonists, may provide targeted therapy for specific subsets of urticaria patients.

Conclusion:

In conclusion, cellular signaling pathways play a crucial role in the pathogenesis of urticaria, regulating inflammation, immune activation, and tissue remodeling. Dysregulation of signaling pathways, including the NF-κB pathway, MAPK pathway, and PI3K/Akt pathway, can lead to excessive inflammation, mast cell activation, and the development of urticarial lesions. Understanding the intricate interplay of cellular signaling pathways in urticaria is essential for elucidating disease mechanisms and identifying potential therapeutic targets. Further research into the regulation and manipulation of signaling pathways may pave the way for more effective treatments for urticaria, improving patient outcomes and quality of life.

Genetic Predisposition in Urticaria

Urticaria, a common dermatological condition characterized by the sudden appearance of wheals, angioedema, and pruritus, has long been recognized to have a multifactorial etiology, with genetic predisposition playing a significant role in disease susceptibility and severity. Genetic factors contribute to the pathogenesis of urticaria through a complex interplay of inherited traits that influence immune responses, inflammatory pathways, and skin barrier function. Understanding the genetic basis of urticaria is essential for elucidating disease mechanisms, identifying genetic risk factors, and developing personalized therapeutic approaches. This comprehensive overview will delve into the multifaceted role of genetic predisposition in urticaria, encompassing genetic risk factors, susceptibility genes, and implications for disease management.

Genetic Risk Factors:

Several genetic risk factors have been implicated in the pathogenesis of urticaria, including polymorphisms in genes encoding proteins involved in immune regulation, inflammatory responses, and skin barrier function. Genetic variants in genes encoding cytokines, chemokines, and their receptors have been associated with altered immune responses and increased susceptibility to urticaria. For example, polymorphisms in the interleukin-4 (IL-4), interleukin-13 (IL-13), and interleukin-10 (IL-10) genes have been linked to allergic and atopic forms of urticaria, highlighting the role of Th2-mediated immune responses in disease pathogenesis. Additionally, genetic variants in genes encoding components of the complement system, such as complement C3 and complement factor H, have been associated with complement-mediated urticaria subtypes, such as urticarial vasculitis and autoimmune urticaria.

Susceptibility Genes:

Genome-wide association studies (GWAS) have identified several susceptibility genes and loci associated with increased risk of urticaria development. These susceptibility genes encompass a wide range of biological processes, including immune regulation, inflammation, and skin barrier function. For example, variants in the gene encoding filaggrin (FLG), a key protein involved in maintaining skin barrier integrity, have been associated with increased susceptibility to chronic spontaneous urticaria (CSU) and atopic dermatitis. Similarly, variants in genes encoding histamine receptors (HRH1, HRH4) and mast cell-associated proteins (KIT, FcεRI) have been linked to mast cell activation and urticaria susceptibility.

Inheritance Patterns:

The inheritance patterns of genetic predisposition in urticaria are complex and may involve both familial aggregation and sporadic mutations. While urticaria often exhibits familial clustering, with an increased risk of disease among first-degree relatives of affected individuals, the inheritance pattern is typically multifactorial and polygenic, involving contributions from multiple genetic and environmental factors. Rare familial forms of urticaria, such as familial cold autoinflammatory syndrome (FCAS) and hereditary angioedema (HAE), result from monogenic mutations in specific genes involved in innate immune pathways or complement regulation, leading to recurrent episodes of urticaria and angioedema.

Implications for Disease Management:

Understanding the genetic basis of urticaria has important implications for disease management and therapeutic intervention. Genetic profiling and risk stratification may help identify individuals at increased risk of developing urticaria or experiencing more severe disease manifestations, enabling targeted screening, surveillance, and early intervention. Additionally, personalized therapeutic approaches based on individual genetic profiles may enhance treatment efficacy and minimize adverse effects by tailoring therapy to specific genetic susceptibilities. For example, genetic testing for polymorphisms in genes encoding drug-metabolizing enzymes or drug transporters may inform drug selection and dosing in patients with urticaria, reducing the risk of adverse drug reactions and treatment failure.

Future Directions:

Future research into the genetic basis of urticaria holds

promise for uncovering novel therapeutic targets and developing precision medicine approaches for disease management. Advances in genomic technologies, such as next-generation sequencing (NGS) and genome editing, may facilitate the identification of rare genetic variants and functional mutations underlying urticaria susceptibility. Integration of genetic data with clinical phenotypes and environmental exposures through large-scale collaborative efforts, such as international consortia and biobanks, may provide insights into gene-environment interactions and personalized risk prediction models for urticaria. Additionally, elucidating the epigenetic mechanisms underlying gene regulation and expression in urticaria may offer new avenues for therapeutic intervention and disease prevention.

Conclusion:

In conclusion, genetic predisposition plays a significant role in the pathogenesis of urticaria, influencing disease susceptibility, severity, and treatment response. Genetic risk factors, susceptibility genes, and inheritance patterns contribute to the complex interplay of immune dysregulation, inflammation, and skin barrier dysfunction underlying urticaria pathophysiology. Understanding the genetic basis of urticaria has important implications for disease management, enabling personalized risk assessment, targeted therapy, and precision medicine approaches. Further research into the genetic determinants of urticaria and their functional significance may pave the way for improved diagnostic tools, novel therapeutic targets, and more effective treatments for this common dermatological condition.

CHAPTER 4: TRIGGERS AND RISK FACTORS

Environmental Triggers in Urticaria

Urticaria, a common dermatological disorder characterized by the sudden onset of wheals, angioedema, and pruritus, is influenced by a myriad of environmental triggers. These triggers encompass a broad spectrum of factors, including allergens, physical stimuli, medications, infections, and emotional stressors, which can precipitate or exacerbate urticarial symptoms in susceptible individuals. Understanding the role of environmental triggers in urticaria is essential for identifying causative factors, implementing preventive measures, and optimizing disease management strategies. This comprehensive overview will explore the diverse array of environmental triggers implicated in urticaria, encompassing allergenic, physical, pharmacological, infectious, and psychological factors.

Allergenic Triggers:

Allergenic triggers represent a common cause of urticaria, particularly in allergic and atopic individuals. Allergens such as pollen, animal dander, dust mites, and food proteins can elicit IgE-mediated immune responses, leading to mast cell activation and the release of inflammatory mediators such as histamine and leukotrienes. Common food allergens implicated in urticaria include nuts, shellfish, eggs, milk, and soy, while inhalant allergens such as pollen, mold spores, and pet dander can trigger allergic rhinitis and urticaria in sensitized individuals. Identification and avoidance of specific allergenic triggers are essential components of managing allergic urticaria, often requiring allergen testing and dietary modifications to minimize symptom exacerbations.

Physical Stimuli:

Physical stimuli represent another significant trigger for urticaria, comprising a diverse range of factors such as temperature changes, pressure, friction, and sunlight exposure. Physical urticaria encompasses various subtypes, including cold urticaria, heat urticaria, pressure urticaria, and solar urticaria, each triggered by specific physical stimuli. Cold urticaria, triggered by exposure to cold temperatures, can manifest as localized or generalized hives following cold exposure, while heat urticaria presents with erythema and wheals upon exposure to warmth. Pressure urticaria typically occurs at sites of sustained pressure or friction, such as tight clothing or prolonged sitting, leading to localized wheals and swelling. Solar urticaria, triggered by sunlight exposure, presents with erythematous lesions and pruritus within minutes of sun exposure, often necessitating photoprotection measures and avoidance of peak sunlight hours.

Pharmacological Triggers:

Medications represent a common cause of urticaria, with numerous drugs implicated in eliciting allergic and non-allergic reactions. Non-steroidal anti-inflammatory drugs (NSAIDs), antibiotics, opioids, angiotensin-converting enzyme (ACE) inhibitors, and radiocontrast agents are among the most frequently reported drug triggers for urticaria. Drug-induced urticaria may result from immune-mediated hypersensitivity reactions, direct mast cell activation, or non-immune mechanisms such as inhibition of cyclooxygenase enzymes or activation of bradykinin pathways. Identifying and avoiding specific medication triggers is essential in managing drug-induced urticaria, often requiring comprehensive medication histories, drug allergy testing, and alternative therapeutic options to minimize adverse reactions.

Infectious Triggers:

Infections, both viral and bacterial, can serve as triggers for acute and chronic urticaria, either through direct immunological mechanisms or as a consequence of immune dysregulation. Viral infections such as upper respiratory tract infections (e.g., common cold), viral exanthems (e.g., Epstein-Barr virus, herpes simplex virus), and viral hepatitis (e.g., hepatitis B and C) have been associated with acute urticarial eruptions, often resolving with viral clearance. Chronic infections such as Helicobacter pylori, hepatitis B and C viruses, and parasitic infestations have been implicated in the pathogenesis of chronic spontaneous urticaria (CSU), with eradication therapy leading to symptom improvement in some cases. Immune-mediated mechanisms, molecular mimicry, and cytokine dysregulation may contribute to the link between infections and urticaria pathogenesis.

Psychological Triggers:

Psychological stressors and emotional factors can exacerbate urticaria symptoms through neuroendocrine and immune-mediated mechanisms, highlighting the complex interplay between the mind and body in disease pathogenesis. Stress-induced urticaria encompasses a spectrum of conditions, including chronic stress-induced urticaria, cholinergic urticaria triggered by emotional stress or physical exertion, and dermatographism exacerbated by psychological stressors. Stress-induced release of cortisol, adrenaline, and neuropeptides can modulate immune responses, mast cell activation, and inflammatory pathways, contributing to urticarial flares in susceptible individuals. Stress management techniques, cognitive-behavioral therapy, and relaxation exercises may help mitigate psychological triggers and improve symptom control in patients with stress-induced urticaria.

Conclusion:

In conclusion, environmental triggers play a pivotal role in the pathogenesis of urticaria, encompassing allergenic, physical, pharmacological, infectious, and psychological factors. Recognition and avoidance of specific triggers are essential components of managing urticaria, often requiring comprehensive patient education, trigger identification, and lifestyle modifications. Multidisciplinary approaches incorporating allergists, dermatologists, immunologists, and psychologists are essential for optimizing disease management strategies and improving patient outcomes. Further research into the mechanisms underlying environmental triggers in urticaria may lead to the development of targeted therapies and personalized interventions tailored to individual trigger profiles, ultimately enhancing the quality of life for patients with this chronic inflammatory skin disorder.

Food Allergens in Urticaria

Urticaria, a common dermatological condition characterized by the sudden appearance of wheals, angioedema, and pruritus, can often be triggered or exacerbated by food allergens. Food allergies represent a significant subset of urticaria cases, particularly in children and individuals with allergic predispositions. Understanding the role of food allergens in urticaria is crucial for identifying causative triggers, implementing dietary modifications, and optimizing disease management strategies. This comprehensive overview will explore the diverse array of food allergens implicated in urticaria, encompassing common allergenic foods, cross-reactive allergens, and diagnostic approaches for identifying food triggers.

Common Food Allergens:

Several common food allergens have been associated with the development of urticaria, including nuts, shellfish, eggs, milk, soy, wheat, and certain fruits and vegetables. These allergenic foods contain proteins that can elicit immune responses in sensitized individuals, leading to mast cell activation and the release of inflammatory mediators such as histamine, leukotrienes, and cytokines. The clinical presentation of food-induced urticaria can vary widely, ranging from localized cutaneous symptoms to systemic reactions such as anaphylaxis, depending on the allergen, route of exposure, and individual sensitivity.

Cross-Reactive Allergens:

Cross-reactivity between allergenic foods and environmental allergens can contribute to the development of food-induced urticaria, particularly in individuals with pollen allergies or latex sensitivities. This phenomenon, known as oral allergy syndrome (OAS) or pollen-food syndrome, occurs when proteins in certain fruits, vegetables, and nuts share structural similarities with pollen or latex allergens, leading to cross-reactive immune responses. For example, individuals allergic to birch pollen may experience oral itching or urticaria upon consuming raw fruits such as apples, pears, and cherries, due to cross-reactivity between birch pollen allergens and fruit proteins.

Diagnostic Approaches:

Diagnosing food-induced urticaria requires a comprehensive clinical evaluation, including detailed patient history, physical examination, and diagnostic testing to identify specific food triggers. Skin prick testing (SPT) and serum-specific IgE testing can help identify allergenic foods by measuring IgE-mediated sensitization to specific food proteins. Oral food challenges, conducted under medical supervision, may be indicated to confirm suspected food allergies or evaluate tolerance to allergenic foods. Additionally, elimination diets and food diaries can help identify trigger foods by tracking symptom exacerbations following food consumption and subsequent reintroduction.

Management Strategies:

Managing food-induced urticaria involves avoiding identified trigger foods, implementing dietary modifications, and providing appropriate treatment for symptom relief and acute reactions. Elimination diets, guided by allergists or dietitians, may involve removing suspected trigger foods from the diet and reintroducing them systematically to identify causative allergens. Label reading and allergen avoidance are essential components of managing food allergies, requiring vigilance in identifying hidden allergens and cross-contamination risks in processed foods. In cases of severe or life-threatening food allergies, carrying self-injectable epinephrine (e.g., EpiPen) and having an emergency action plan in place are critical for managing anaphylactic reactions.

Future Directions:

Future research into food allergens and their role in urticaria pathogenesis holds promise for advancing diagnostic methods, identifying novel allergenic proteins, and developing targeted therapies for food-induced urticaria. Advances in allergen component testing, utilizing purified proteins and molecular diagnostics, may improve the accuracy and specificity of allergy testing, particularly in cases of cross-reactive allergens and polysensitization. Additionally, allergen-specific immunotherapy (AIT) for food allergies, such as oral immunotherapy (OIT) and sublingual immunotherapy (SLIT), may offer potential treatment options for desensitizing individuals to specific food allergens and reducing allergic reactions.

Conclusion:

In conclusion, food allergens play a significant role in the pathogenesis of urticaria, contributing to mast cell activation, inflammation, and symptom exacerbations in susceptible individuals. Identifying and avoiding specific food triggers are essential components of managing food-induced urticaria, requiring comprehensive diagnostic evaluation, allergen testing, and dietary modifications. Cross-reactive allergens and environmental sensitivities further complicate the diagnosis and management of food allergies, necessitating a multidisciplinary approach involving allergists, dermatologists, dietitians, and other healthcare professionals. Future research into food allergens and their interactions with the immune system may lead to improved diagnostic methods, personalized treatment approaches, and enhanced quality of life for patients with food-induced urticaria.

Medications Associated with Urticaria

Urticaria, a common dermatological condition characterized by the sudden onset of wheals, angioedema, and pruritus, can often be triggered or exacerbated by various medications. Drug-induced urticaria represents a significant subset of urticaria cases, encompassing a diverse array of pharmaceutical agents that can elicit allergic and non-allergic reactions in susceptible individuals. Understanding the medications associated with urticaria is crucial for identifying potential triggers, implementing preventive measures, and optimizing disease management strategies. This comprehensive overview will explore the diverse range of medications implicated in urticaria, encompassing common drug classes, mechanisms of drug-induced urticaria, and diagnostic approaches for identifying medication triggers.

Common Medications Associated with Urticaria:

Numerous medications have been reported to induce urticarial reactions, including non-steroidal anti-inflammatory drugs (NSAIDs), antibiotics, opioids, angiotensin-converting enzyme (ACE) inhibitors, radiocontrast agents, and biologic therapies. NSAIDs, such as aspirin, ibuprofen, and naproxen, are among the most frequently reported drug triggers for urticaria, often causing non-immune-mediated reactions through inhibition of cyclooxygenase enzymes and subsequent release of inflammatory mediators. Antibiotics, particularly beta-lactams (e.g., penicillins, cephalosporins) and sulfonamides, can elicit allergic reactions, including urticaria, through drug-specific IgE-mediated mechanisms or non-immune pathways. Opioids, such as morphine and codeine, may induce urticaria via direct histamine release or immune-mediated hypersensitivity reactions.

Mechanisms of Drug-Induced Urticaria:

Drug-induced urticaria can result from various immunological and non-immunological mechanisms, depending on the specific drug, patient characteristics, and underlying predispositions. Immunological mechanisms involve drug-specific IgE-mediated hypersensitivity reactions, characterized by the formation of drug-specific IgE antibodies and subsequent mast cell activation upon re-exposure to the offending drug. Non-immunological mechanisms, such as direct mast cell degranulation, complement activation, or pharmacological effects on histamine release, may also contribute to drug-induced urticarial reactions. Additionally, non-specific factors such as dose-related effects, drug metabolism, and individual susceptibility may influence the likelihood and severity of drug-induced urticaria.

Diagnostic Approaches:

Diagnosing drug-induced urticaria requires a thorough clinical evaluation, including detailed patient history, physical examination, and diagnostic testing to identify potential medication triggers. Patient-reported symptoms, including timing of symptom onset relative to drug exposure, duration of symptoms, and presence of associated symptoms such as angioedema or anaphylaxis, can provide valuable clues to potential drug-induced reactions. Skin prick testing (SPT) and serum-specific IgE testing may be indicated to assess for IgE-mediated sensitization to specific drug allergens, particularly in cases of suspected antibiotic allergies. Drug provocation testing (DPT), conducted under medical supervision, may be required to confirm suspected drug allergies or evaluate tolerance to specific medications.

Management Strategies:

Managing drug-induced urticaria involves identifying and avoiding implicated medications, implementing alternative treatment options, and providing appropriate symptomatic relief for acute reactions. In cases of suspected drug allergies, consultation with an allergist or immunologist is recommended to confirm diagnoses, identify cross-reactive drug allergens, and develop personalized treatment plans. Medication reconciliation and comprehensive drug allergy documentation are essential components of managing drug-induced urticaria, requiring collaboration between healthcare providers, pharmacists, and patients to minimize the risk of inadvertent drug exposures and adverse reactions.

Future Directions:

Future research into drug-induced urticaria holds promise for advancing diagnostic methods, elucidating underlying mechanisms, and developing targeted therapies for specific drug allergies. Advances in drug allergy testing, including component-resolved diagnostics and basophil activation testing, may improve the accuracy and specificity of drug allergy diagnosis, particularly in cases of non-IgE-mediated reactions or cross-reactive drug allergens. Additionally, pharmacogenomic approaches may help identify genetic risk factors for drug-induced urticaria, enabling personalized treatment strategies and minimizing adverse drug reactions.

Conclusion:

In conclusion, medications represent a significant trigger for urticaria, encompassing a diverse range of pharmaceutical agents that can elicit allergic and non-allergic reactions in susceptible individuals. Understanding the medications associated with urticaria is essential for identifying potential triggers, implementing preventive measures, and optimizing disease management strategies. Comprehensive clinical evaluation, diagnostic testing, and collaboration between healthcare providers are essential for diagnosing and managing drug-induced urticaria effectively. Further research into the mechanisms and management of drug-induced urticaria may lead to improved diagnostic methods, personalized treatment approaches, and enhanced patient outcomes in the future.

Physical Triggers in Urticaria: Understanding Cold, Heat, Pressure, and More

Urticaria, a dermatological condition characterized by the sudden appearance of wheals, angioedema, and pruritus, can be triggered or exacerbated by various physical factors. These physical triggers encompass a diverse range of stimuli, including cold, heat, pressure, vibration, and friction, which can induce urticarial reactions in susceptible individuals. Understanding the role of physical triggers in urticaria is crucial for identifying causative factors, implementing preventive measures, and optimizing disease management strategies. This comprehensive overview will explore the diverse array of physical triggers implicated in urticaria, encompassing cold-induced urticaria, heat-induced urticaria, pressure urticaria, and other related conditions.

Cold-Induced Urticaria:

Cold-induced urticaria is characterized by the development of wheals and itching upon exposure to cold temperatures, ranging from mild cold urticaria to more severe forms such as cold-induced anaphylaxis. Cold urticaria can occur following exposure to cold air, water, or cold objects, leading to localized or generalized urticarial reactions within minutes of exposure. Severe cases of cold urticaria may result in systemic symptoms such as hypotension, syncope, or anaphylaxis, requiring prompt medical attention. Management of cold-induced urticaria involves avoiding cold exposure, wearing protective clothing, and using antihistamines or epinephrine as needed for symptom relief.

Heat-Induced Urticaria:

Heat-induced urticaria, also known as cholinergic urticaria, is characterized by the development of small, pinpoint wheals and itching in response to increased body temperature, sweating, or physical exertion. Cholinergic urticaria typically occurs during or after activities that induce sweating, such as exercise, hot showers, or emotional stress, leading to transient urticarial lesions and pruritus. The pathogenesis of cholinergic urticaria involves activation of sweat gland acetylcholine receptors, leading to mast cell degranulation and histamine release. Management of heat-induced urticaria may involve avoiding triggers, staying cool, and using antihistamines or anticholinergic agents for symptom relief.

Pressure Urticaria:

Pressure urticaria is characterized by the development of wheals and swelling at sites of sustained pressure or friction, such as tight clothing, belts, or straps. Pressure urticaria typically presents as localized erythematous lesions, swelling, and tenderness at pressure points, often persisting for hours to days after the removal of pressure stimuli. The pathogenesis of pressure urticaria involves mechanical trauma to dermal mast cells, leading to histamine release and inflammatory responses. Management of pressure urticaria may involve avoiding tight clothing, using protective padding, and using antihistamines or corticosteroids for symptom relief.

Vibration-Induced Urticaria:

Vibration-induced urticaria is a rare form of physical urticaria characterized by the development of wheals and itching in response to mechanical vibration or friction, such as using power tools, riding motorcycles, or operating vibrating machinery. Vibration urticaria typically presents as localized or generalized wheals and erythematous lesions at sites of vibratory exposure, accompanied by pruritus and discomfort. The pathogenesis of vibration urticaria involves mechanical stimulation of dermal mast cells, leading to histamine release and inflammatory responses. Management of vibration-induced urticaria may involve avoiding vibratory stimuli, using protective equipment, and using antihistamines or corticosteroids for symptom relief.

Aquagenic Urticaria:

Aquagenic urticaria is a rare form of physical urticaria characterized by the development of wheals and itching upon contact with water, regardless of temperature or source. Aquagenic urticaria typically presents as localized or generalized erythematous lesions and pruritus within minutes of water exposure, often resolving within 30-60 minutes after drying. The pathogenesis of aquagenic urticaria remains poorly understood, with proposed mechanisms including water-induced mast cell degranulation, altered skin barrier function, or osmotic changes in the skin. Management of aquagenic urticaria may involve minimizing water contact, using protective barriers such as waterproof clothing or gloves, and using antihistamines or corticosteroids for symptom relief.

Conclusion:

In conclusion, physical triggers play a significant role in the pathogenesis of urticaria, encompassing a diverse range of stimuli such as cold, heat, pressure, vibration, and water. Understanding the mechanisms underlying physical urticaria is essential for identifying causative factors, implementing preventive measures, and optimizing disease management strategies. Management of physical urticaria involves avoiding trigger stimuli, using protective measures, and using pharmacological therapies for symptom relief. Further research into the pathogenesis and management of physical urticaria may lead to improved diagnostic methods, targeted therapies, and enhanced quality of life for patients with this chronic inflammatory skin disorder.

Stress and Psychological Factors in Urticaria: Understanding the Mind-Body Connection

Urticaria, a common dermatological condition characterized by the sudden appearance of wheals, angioedema, and pruritus, is intricately linked to stress and psychological factors. Stress-induced urticaria encompasses a spectrum of conditions, including acute stress-induced urticaria, chronic stress-induced urticaria, and psychogenic urticaria, which are triggered or exacerbated by emotional stressors, psychological distress, and neuroendocrine responses. Understanding the complex interplay between stress and urticaria is crucial for identifying triggers, implementing stress management techniques, and optimizing disease management strategies. This comprehensive overview will explore the multifaceted relationship between stress, psychological factors, and urticaria, encompassing the neurobiological mechanisms, psychosocial stressors, and therapeutic interventions involved.

Neurobiological Mechanisms:

The neurobiological mechanisms underlying stress-induced urticaria involve complex interactions between the central nervous system, neuroendocrine pathways, and immune responses. Stress activates the hypothalamic-pituitary-adrenal (HPA) axis, leading to the release of stress hormones such as cortisol and adrenaline, which modulate immune function, inflammation, and skin barrier integrity. Cortisol exerts anti-inflammatory effects by suppressing cytokine production, inhibiting mast cell activation, and regulating immune responses, whereas adrenaline stimulates mast cell degranulation and histamine release, contributing to urticarial symptoms. Dysregulation of the HPA axis, alterations in stress hormone levels, and impaired stress coping mechanisms may predispose individuals to stress-induced urticaria.

Psychosocial Stressors:

Psychosocial stressors, including life events, interpersonal conflicts, work-related stress, and emotional distress, can precipitate or exacerbate urticarial symptoms through neuroendocrine and immune-mediated pathways. Acute stressors such as traumatic events, deadlines, or public speaking engagements may trigger acute stress-induced urticaria, leading to transient exacerbations of urticarial lesions and pruritus. Chronic stressors such as ongoing relationship problems, financial difficulties, or caregiving responsibilities may contribute to the development of chronic stress-induced urticaria, characterized by persistent or recurrent urticarial symptoms. Additionally, psychological factors such as anxiety, depression, and perceived stress may exacerbate urticaria through psychosomatic mechanisms, influencing symptom severity and treatment outcomes.

Psychogenic Urticaria:

Psychogenic urticaria, also known as somatoform urticaria or psychosomatic urticaria, refers to urticarial symptoms that are primarily or solely attributable to psychological factors, without evidence of organic pathology or allergic triggers. Psychogenic urticaria is often associated with underlying psychiatric conditions such as somatoform disorders, conversion disorders, or anxiety disorders, where emotional distress or unresolved psychological conflicts manifest as physical symptoms. Psychogenic urticaria may present with atypical clinical features, such as variable lesion morphology, inconsistent triggers, and poor response to conventional treatments, highlighting the importance of psychological assessment and intervention in managing these cases.

Therapeutic Interventions:

Managing stress-induced urticaria involves addressing both the physical symptoms of urticaria and the underlying psychological factors contributing to symptom exacerbations. Multidisciplinary approaches incorporating dermatologists, psychologists, and psychiatrists are essential for optimizing disease management strategies and improving patient outcomes. Stress management techniques, such as relaxation exercises, mindfulness meditation, biofeedback, and cognitive-behavioral therapy (CBT), can help individuals cope with stressors, reduce anxiety levels, and mitigate urticarial symptoms. Psychiatric interventions, including pharmacotherapy with selective serotonin reuptake inhibitors (SSRIs), anxiolytics, or antidepressants, may be indicated for individuals with comorbid psychiatric disorders or severe psychogenic urticaria.

Conclusion:

In conclusion, stress and psychological factors play a significant role in the pathogenesis of urticaria, influencing disease susceptibility, symptom exacerbations, and treatment outcomes. Understanding the complex interplay between stress, neuroendocrine responses, and immune-mediated mechanisms is crucial for identifying triggers, implementing stress management techniques, and optimizing disease management strategies. Multidisciplinary approaches incorporating dermatological, psychological, and psychiatric interventions are essential for addressing both the physical and psychological aspects of urticaria. Further research into the neurobiological mechanisms, psychosocial stressors, and therapeutic interventions for stress-induced urticaria may lead to improved diagnostic methods, targeted therapies, and enhanced quality of life for patients with this chronic inflammatory skin disorder.

CHAPTER 5: DIFFERENTIAL DIAGNOSIS

Distinguishing Chronic Hives from Acute Urticaria: Understanding the Clinical and Pathophysiological Differences

Urticaria, a common dermatological condition characterized by the sudden appearance of wheals, angioedema, and pruritus, encompasses a spectrum of clinical presentations, ranging from acute, self-limited episodes to chronic, persistent symptoms. Distinguishing between chronic hives and acute urticaria is essential for appropriate diagnosis, treatment selection, and management strategies. This comprehensive overview will explore the clinical features, underlying pathophysiology, diagnostic criteria, and management considerations that differentiate chronic hives from acute urticaria, providing insights into their distinct characteristics and implications for patient care.

Clinical Features:

Acute urticaria is defined as the sudden onset of urticarial lesions lasting less than six weeks, typically characterized by transient wheals and pruritus triggered by allergens, infections, medications, or physical stimuli. Acute urticaria often resolves spontaneously within hours to days, with or without treatment, and may recur intermittently in response to ongoing exposures. In contrast, chronic hives, also known as chronic spontaneous urticaria (CSU), is characterized by the recurrent or persistent presence of urticarial lesions lasting six weeks or longer, occurring daily or almost daily, without identifiable triggers. Chronic hives may be associated with significant morbidity, impairment of quality of life, and psychological distress due to the unpredictable nature of symptoms and lack of resolution.

Underlying Pathophysiology:

The underlying pathophysiology of chronic hives and acute urticaria differs in terms of immune dysregulation, inflammatory mediators, and disease mechanisms. Acute urticaria is often triggered by IgE-mediated immune responses to specific allergens, leading to mast cell activation, histamine release, and transient urticarial lesions. Common triggers for acute urticaria include food allergies, insect stings, medications, infections, and physical stimuli. In contrast, chronic hives are characterized by a dysregulated immune response involving autoantibodies against mast cell or basophil surface receptors, such as IgE or IgG, leading to chronic mast cell activation and sustained release of inflammatory mediators. Autoimmune mechanisms, complement activation, and neurogenic factors may contribute to the pathogenesis of chronic hives, resulting in persistent urticarial symptoms despite the absence of identifiable triggers.

Diagnostic Criteria:

The diagnosis of chronic hives and acute urticaria is primarily based on clinical history, physical examination, and characteristic skin findings, with additional diagnostic testing to identify underlying triggers or associated conditions. Chronic hives are defined by the presence of urticarial lesions lasting six weeks or longer, occurring daily or almost daily, without identifiable triggers, based on established diagnostic criteria such as the EAACI/GA^{2}LEN/EDF/WAO guidelines. Diagnostic evaluation for chronic hives may include laboratory testing to assess for autoimmune markers (e.g., anti-IgE receptor antibodies, anti-thyroid antibodies), complement levels, and inflammatory markers. In contrast, acute urticaria is diagnosed based on the sudden onset of urticarial lesions lasting less than six weeks, often associated with identifiable triggers such as allergens, infections, medications, or physical stimuli. Diagnostic testing for acute urticaria may include allergy testing, infectious disease screening, and medication histories to identify potential triggers.

Management Considerations:

Management strategies for chronic hives and acute urticaria differ in terms of treatment goals, therapeutic interventions, and follow-up monitoring. Acute urticaria may be managed with symptomatic relief using oral antihistamines, corticosteroids, or other pharmacological agents to alleviate itching and reduce inflammation. Identifying and avoiding specific triggers for acute urticaria is essential for preventing symptom recurrence and optimizing treatment outcomes. In contrast, chronic hives often require long-term management with second-generation H1 antihistamines as first-line therapy, with additional treatment options such as omalizumab, cyclosporine, or immunomodulatory agents for refractory cases. Monitoring disease activity, assessing treatment response, and adjusting therapy based on individual patient needs are essential components of managing chronic hives.

Conclusion:

In conclusion, distinguishing between chronic hives and acute urticaria is essential for accurate diagnosis, appropriate treatment selection, and optimal management strategies. While both conditions share common clinical features such as wheals, angioedema, and pruritus, their underlying pathophysiology, diagnostic criteria, and management considerations differ significantly. Understanding the distinct characteristics of chronic hives and acute urticaria is essential for healthcare providers to provide comprehensive care and improve patient outcomes. Further research into the pathogenesis, diagnostic approaches, and treatment options for chronic hives and acute urticaria may lead to advancements in disease management and personalized therapeutic strategies for patients with these debilitating skin disorders.

Exploring Other Causes of Persistent Rash: Differential Diagnosis and Clinical Considerations

While chronic hives and acute urticaria represent common etiologies of persistent rash, several other underlying conditions must be considered in the differential diagnosis. This comprehensive overview will explore the diverse array of potential causes of persistent rash beyond chronic hives and acute urticaria, encompassing dermatological, infectious, autoimmune, and systemic disorders. Understanding these alternative etiologies is crucial for accurate diagnosis, appropriate treatment selection, and optimal management strategies.

Dermatological Conditions:

Numerous dermatological conditions can present with persistent rash, including eczema (atopic dermatitis), psoriasis, contact dermatitis, seborrheic dermatitis, and drug eruptions. Eczema is characterized by pruritic, erythematous patches with a predilection for flexural surfaces, often associated with a personal or family history of allergic diseases. Psoriasis presents with well-demarcated, erythematous plaques covered with silvery scales, typically involving extensor surfaces, scalp, and nails. Contact dermatitis results from exposure to irritants or allergens, leading to erythema, vesicles, and pruritus at the site of contact. Seborrheic dermatitis manifests as erythematous, greasy scales on the scalp, face, and trunk, often associated with yeast overgrowth. Drug eruptions can result from adverse reactions to medications, presenting with various morphologies, including maculopapular rash, urticaria, or exfoliative dermatitis.

Infectious Causes:

Infectious agents, including bacteria, viruses, fungi, and parasites, can cause persistent rash through direct skin invasion, immune-mediated reactions, or toxin production. Bacterial infections such as cellulitis, impetigo, folliculitis, and erysipelas can present with erythematous, tender plaques, pustules, or vesicles, often accompanied by fever and systemic symptoms. Viral infections such as herpes simplex virus (HSV), varicella-zoster virus (VZV), human herpesvirus 6 (HHV-6), and cytomegalovirus (CMV) can cause vesicular or pustular rashes, with characteristic distribution patterns and associated symptoms. Fungal infections such as tinea corporis (ringworm), candidiasis, and pityriasis versicolor can present with erythematous, scaly patches, or plaques, often associated with pruritus and fungal cultures. Parasitic infestations such as scabies and lice can cause pruritic papules, burrows, or nodules, typically involving intertriginous areas, wrists, and genitalia.

Autoimmune Disorders:

Autoimmune disorders involving the skin can present with persistent rash as a primary or secondary manifestation of immune dysregulation. Conditions such as lupus erythematosus (LE), dermatomyositis, systemic sclerosis, and autoimmune blistering diseases (e.g., pemphigus, bullous pemphigoid) can present with cutaneous manifestations ranging from maculopapular rash and erythema to vesicles, bullae, and erosions. LE can present with various subtypes, including acute cutaneous LE (ACLE), subacute cutaneous LE (SCLE), and chronic cutaneous LE (CCLE), each with distinct clinical and histological features. Dermatomyositis is characterized by heliotrope rash (violaceous erythema on the eyelids), Gottron's papules (erythematous papules overlying bony prominences), and proximal muscle weakness. Systemic sclerosis can present with sclerodactyly, Raynaud's phenomenon, digital ulcers, and telangiectasias, with variable cutaneous involvement.

Systemic Diseases:

Several systemic diseases can manifest with cutaneous findings, including endocrine disorders, hematologic malignancies, rheumatologic diseases, and metabolic disorders. Endocrine disorders such as thyroid dysfunction (hypothyroidism, hyperthyroidism), adrenal insufficiency (Addison's disease), and diabetes mellitus (diabetic dermopathy) can present with various cutaneous manifestations, including dry skin, alopecia, skin thickening, and diabetic neuropathy. Hematologic malignancies such as leukemia, lymphoma, and myeloproliferative disorders can present with cutaneous involvement, including leukemia cutis, lymphomatous infiltrates, and paraneoplastic syndromes. Rheumatologic diseases such as rheumatoid arthritis, systemic lupus erythematosus (SLE), and systemic vasculitis can cause various cutaneous manifestations, including rheumatoid nodules, malar rash, and livedo reticularis. Metabolic disorders such as amyloidosis, porphyria, and Fabry disease can present with characteristic cutaneous findings, including purpura, blistering, and angiokeratomas.

Conclusion:

In conclusion, several alternative etiologies must be considered in the differential diagnosis of persistent rash beyond chronic hives and acute urticaria. Dermatological conditions, infectious causes, autoimmune disorders, and systemic diseases can all present with cutaneous manifestations, necessitating a comprehensive clinical evaluation, diagnostic workup, and multidisciplinary approach to patient care. Identifying the underlying cause of persistent rash is crucial for appropriate treatment selection, management strategies, and patient outcomes. Further research into the pathogenesis, diagnostic criteria, and therapeutic interventions for various cutaneous conditions may lead to advancements in disease management and personalized treatment approaches for patients with persistent rash.

Understanding Urticarial Vasculitis: Clinical Features, Pathogenesis, Diagnosis, and Management

Urticarial vasculitis (UV) is a rare form of vasculitis characterized by the presence of urticarial lesions with histopathological evidence of leukocytoclastic vasculitis. While UV shares some clinical features with ordinary urticaria, it is distinguished by its chronicity, persistence, and potential for systemic involvement. This comprehensive overview will explore the clinical features, underlying pathogenesis, diagnostic criteria, and management considerations of urticarial vasculitis, providing insights into this rare but significant dermatological condition.

Clinical Features:

Urticarial vasculitis typically presents with urticarial lesions that are indistinguishable from those seen in ordinary urticaria, including erythematous wheals, pruritus, and occasionally angioedema. However, unlike ordinary urticaria, urticarial vasculitis lesions persist for more than 24 hours and often leave residual purpura or hyperpigmentation upon resolution. UV lesions may exhibit a fixed distribution pattern, tenderness, and burning sensation, distinguishing them from transient, migratory wheals of ordinary urticaria. Systemic symptoms such as arthralgia, myalgia, fever, and constitutional symptoms may occur in a subset of patients, reflecting systemic inflammation and immune dysregulation.

Pathogenesis:

The pathogenesis of urticarial vasculitis involves immune-mediated inflammation and small vessel vasculitis, leading to the characteristic histopathological findings of leukocytoclastic vasculitis. Immune complexes, complement activation, and endothelial injury contribute to vascular inflammation, neutrophil infiltration, and fibrinoid necrosis within the vessel walls. The exact triggers and underlying mechanisms of UV remain incompletely understood, although autoimmune processes, hypersensitivity reactions, and complement dysregulation have been implicated in disease pathogenesis. In some cases, UV may be associated with underlying systemic diseases such as systemic lupus erythematosus (SLE), connective tissue disorders, autoimmune hepatitis, or malignancies, highlighting the importance of comprehensive evaluation and disease screening.

Diagnosis:

The diagnosis of urticarial vasculitis relies on clinical evaluation, characteristic histopathological findings, and exclusion of other causes of chronic urticaria. Skin biopsy of lesional skin demonstrates leukocytoclastic vasculitis, characterized by neutrophilic infiltrates, fibrinoid necrosis, and vascular damage in the small vessels of the dermis. Direct immunofluorescence (DIF) microscopy may reveal immune complex deposition along the vessel walls, supporting the diagnosis of UV. Laboratory evaluation may include complete blood count (CBC), erythrocyte sedimentation rate (ESR), C-reactive protein (CRP), serum complement levels (C3, C4), antinuclear antibodies (ANA), and specific autoantibodies (e.g., anti-nuclear cytoplasmic antibodies, anti-double-stranded DNA antibodies) to assess for underlying systemic diseases or immune dysregulation.

DR. SPINEANUEUGENIA

Management:

The management of urticarial vasculitis involves symptomatic relief, disease control, and treatment of underlying systemic conditions. Non-steroidal anti-inflammatory drugs (NSAIDs), antihistamines, and corticosteroids are commonly used for symptomatic relief of pruritus, inflammation, and angioedema associated with UV lesions. Topical corticosteroids may be effective for localized lesions, while systemic corticosteroids are reserved for more severe or refractory cases. Immunomodulatory agents such as hydroxychloroquine, colchicine, dapsone, or azathioprine may be considered for long-term disease control and steroid-sparing effects. In cases of UV associated with underlying systemic diseases, treatment should be directed at controlling the underlying condition, addressing autoimmune inflammation, and preventing disease progression.

Prognosis:

The prognosis of urticarial vasculitis varies depending on the underlying etiology, disease severity, and response to treatment. While some patients may experience spontaneous remission or mild disease course, others may develop chronic, relapsing disease with systemic complications. Long-term follow-up is essential to monitor disease activity, assess treatment response, and detect potential complications such as systemic involvement, organ damage, or malignancies. Close collaboration between dermatologists, rheumatologists, and other specialists is crucial for comprehensive management and optimal outcomes in patients with urticarial vasculitis.

Conclusion:

In conclusion, urticarial vasculitis is a rare but significant form of vasculitis characterized by chronic urticarial lesions with evidence of leukocytoclastic vasculitis on histopathology. Clinical recognition, appropriate diagnostic evaluation, and comprehensive management are essential for effectively managing urticarial vasculitis and preventing disease-related complications. Further research into the pathogenesis, biomarkers, and targeted therapies for urticarial vasculitis may lead to advancements in disease understanding and personalized treatment approaches for this challenging dermatological condition.

Understanding Dermatographic Urticaria: Clinical Features, Mechanisms, Diagnosis, and Management

Dermatographic urticaria, also known as dermographism or skin writing, is a common form of physical urticaria characterized by the development of linear wheals or welts in response to physical pressure or stroking of the skin. While dermatographic urticaria is typically benign and self-limiting, it can cause significant discomfort and impairment of quality of life in affected individuals. This comprehensive overview will explore the clinical features, underlying mechanisms, diagnostic criteria, and management strategies of dermatographic urticaria, providing insights into this unique dermatological condition.

Clinical Features:

Dermatographic urticaria presents with the characteristic appearance of linear wheals or welts (wheals) that develop rapidly following mechanical stimulation of the skin, such as scratching, rubbing, or pressure from clothing or objects. The wheals typically appear within minutes of skin stimulation and may persist for 30 minutes to several hours before resolving spontaneously. The wheals are typically erythematous or pink in color, raised, and pruritic, often following the pattern of the applied pressure or scratching. In severe cases, extensive scratching or rubbing may lead to the formation of large, confluent wheals or localized angioedema, causing significant discomfort and distress.

Mechanisms:

The underlying mechanisms of dermatographic urticaria involve mast cell activation and histamine release in response to mechanical stimulation of the skin. Mast cells, which are abundant in the dermis, contain granules filled with inflammatory mediators such as histamine, leukotrienes, and prostaglandins. Mechanical pressure or friction on the skin triggers degranulation of mast cells, leading to the release of these inflammatory mediators into the surrounding tissue. Histamine, in particular, causes vasodilation, increased vascular permeability, and activation of sensory nerve fibers, resulting in the characteristic wheal and flare response seen in dermatographic urticaria. Other mediators such as leukotrienes and prostaglandins may also contribute to the inflammatory response and pruritus associated with dermatographic urticaria.

Diagnosis:

The diagnosis of dermatographic urticaria is primarily based on clinical history, physical examination, and characteristic skin findings. The demonstration of a dermatographism response, characterized by the development of wheals or welts following firm stroking or scratching of the skin, is a hallmark feature of dermatographic urticaria. Skin testing with a blunt object or fingernail may be performed to elicit a dermatographism response and confirm the diagnosis. Laboratory testing is generally not required for the diagnosis of dermatographic urticaria unless other underlying conditions are suspected. Differential diagnosis may include other forms of physical urticaria, such as pressure urticaria, cold urticaria, or cholinergic urticaria, which may present with similar clinical features.

Management:

The management of dermatographic urticaria focuses on symptom relief, minimizing triggers, and preventing exacerbations of symptoms. Avoidance of friction, pressure, or scratching of the skin is essential for preventing the development of wheals and minimizing pruritus. Loose-fitting clothing made from soft, breathable fabrics may help reduce skin irritation and friction. Topical emollients or moisturizers can help maintain skin barrier function and reduce dryness and irritation. Oral antihistamines, such as second-generation H1 antihistamines (e.g., cetirizine, loratadine, fexofenadine), are the mainstay of pharmacological therapy for dermatographic urticaria, providing symptomatic relief of pruritus and reducing mast cell activation. In severe or refractory cases, short-term use of oral corticosteroids may be considered for rapid symptom control, although long-term use should be avoided due to potential side effects.

Prognosis:

The prognosis of dermatographic urticaria is generally favorable, with most cases resolving spontaneously or responding well to conservative management strategies. While dermatographic urticaria can cause significant discomfort and impairment of quality of life, it is not associated with systemic complications or long-term health effects. With appropriate avoidance of triggers and use of symptomatic treatments, most individuals with dermatographic urticaria can achieve good control of their symptoms and lead normal lives.

Conclusion:

In conclusion, dermatographic urticaria is a common form of physical urticaria characterized by the development of linear wheals or welts in response to mechanical stimulation of the skin. Understanding the clinical features, underlying mechanisms, diagnostic criteria, and management strategies of dermatographic urticaria is essential for accurate diagnosis, appropriate treatment selection, and optimal patient care. Further research into the pathophysiology, genetic predisposition, and targeted therapies for dermatographic urticaria may lead to advancements in disease understanding and personalized treatment approaches for individuals affected by this unique dermatological condition.

CHAPTER 6: CLINICAL MANAGEMENT

Pharmacological Treatment Options for Urticaria: A Comprehensive Review

Urticaria, characterized by the sudden appearance of wheals, angioedema, and pruritus, can significantly impact patients' quality of life. Pharmacological interventions play a crucial role in managing urticaria, aiming to alleviate symptoms, suppress inflammation, and improve patient outcomes. This comprehensive review will explore the pharmacological treatment options for urticaria, including antihistamines, leukotriene antagonists, corticosteroids, and immunomodulators, highlighting their mechanisms of action, efficacy, adverse effects, and clinical considerations.

Pharmacological Treatment Options

Pharmacological management of urticaria encompasses a variety of agents targeting different pathways involved in the pathogenesis of the disease. These agents include antihistamines, leukotriene antagonists, corticosteroids, and immunomodulators, each offering unique benefits and considerations in the management of urticaria.

Antihistamines

Antihistamines are the first-line treatment for urticaria, exerting their therapeutic effects by blocking histamine receptors and inhibiting the actions of histamine, a key mediator of urticarial symptoms. First-generation antihistamines, such as diphenhydramine and hydroxyzine, possess sedative properties due to their ability to cross the blood-brain barrier and exert central nervous system effects. Second-generation antihistamines, including cetirizine, loratadine, and fexofenadine, are preferred for their non-sedating properties and reduced risk of cognitive impairment.

The efficacy of antihistamines in the treatment of urticaria has been well-established through numerous clinical trials and real-world studies. These agents effectively reduce pruritus, suppress the formation of wheals, and improve overall disease control in patients with acute and chronic urticaria. Second-generation antihistamines are recommended as first-line therapy due to their favorable safety profile, once-daily dosing, and minimal sedative effects, making them suitable for long-term use.

Leukotriene Antagonists

Leukotriene antagonists, such as montelukast and zafirlukast, target the leukotriene pathway, which plays a role in the pathogenesis of chronic urticaria. Leukotrienes are inflammatory mediators released by mast cells and other immune cells, contributing to vascular permeability, inflammation, and pruritus. By blocking the action of leukotrienes, leukotriene antagonists help reduce inflammation and improve symptoms in patients with chronic urticaria.

While leukotriene antagonists have shown efficacy in some patients with chronic urticaria, their role in the management of the disease remains controversial. Clinical trials investigating the use of leukotriene antagonists as monotherapy or adjunctive therapy in chronic urticaria have yielded mixed results, with some studies demonstrating modest benefits in symptom control and others showing no significant difference compared to placebo. As such, leukotriene antagonists are not considered first-line therapy for urticaria but may be considered as an adjunctive treatment option in patients who are refractory to antihistamines or corticosteroids.

Corticosteroids

Corticosteroids, such as prednisone and prednisolone, exert potent anti-inflammatory effects by suppressing immune responses, inhibiting cytokine production, and reducing vascular permeability. While corticosteroids can effectively alleviate symptoms of urticaria, their use is generally limited to short-term or acute situations due to the risk of adverse effects associated with long-term use, including immunosuppression, osteoporosis, and metabolic disturbances.

In the management of urticaria, corticosteroids are typically reserved for severe, refractory cases or acute exacerbations requiring rapid symptom control. Short courses of oral corticosteroids may be prescribed for acute episodes of urticaria to achieve rapid resolution of symptoms, followed by tapering to minimize the risk of rebound flare-ups and adverse effects. Long-term use of corticosteroids is generally discouraged in chronic urticaria due to the risk of systemic complications and the availability of safer, more effective treatment options.

Immunomodulators

Immunomodulators, such as cyclosporine, methotrexate, and omalizumab, target immune dysregulation and inflammatory pathways implicated in the pathogenesis of chronic urticaria. These agents modulate immune responses, inhibit cytokine production, and suppress inflammatory mediators, offering alternative treatment options for patients with refractory or severe urticaria unresponsive to conventional therapies.

Omalizumab, a monoclonal antibody targeting IgE, has emerged as a promising therapeutic option for chronic urticaria. By binding to free IgE and preventing its interaction with mast cells and basophils, omalizumab inhibits the release of inflammatory mediators and attenuates urticarial symptoms. Clinical trials have demonstrated the efficacy and safety of omalizumab in reducing symptom severity, improving quality of life, and achieving long-term disease control in patients with chronic spontaneous urticaria refractory to antihistamines.

Cyclosporine, an immunosuppressive agent, has also been used off-label in the treatment of chronic urticaria, particularly in patients with severe, recalcitrant disease. Cyclosporine modulates T-cell activation and cytokine production, leading to suppression of immune responses and reduction of inflammatory mediators. While effective in some patients, cyclosporine carries the risk of significant adverse effects, including nephrotoxicity, hypertension, and opportunistic infections, necessitating close monitoring and careful risk-benefit assessment.

Methotrexate, a folic acid antagonist, has been investigated as an alternative treatment option for chronic urticaria, particularly in patients with autoimmune or inflammatory subtypes of the disease. Methotrexate exerts immunosuppressive and anti-inflammatory effects by inhibiting purine and pyrimidine synthesis, suppressing lymphocyte proliferation, and reducing cytokine production. While methotrexate may offer benefits in selected patients, its use is limited by potential hepatotoxicity, bone marrow suppression, and gastrointestinal side effects, requiring careful monitoring and dose adjustments.

Conclusion

In conclusion, pharmacological treatment options for urticaria encompass a variety of agents targeting different pathways involved in the pathogenesis of the disease. Antihistamines are the mainstay of therapy for urticaria, providing symptomatic relief and improving disease control in most patients. Leukotriene antagonists, corticosteroids, and immunomodulators offer additional treatment options for patients with refractory or severe urticaria unresponsive to conventional therapies. Individualized treatment approaches, taking into account disease severity, subtype, comorbidities, and patient preferences, are essential for optimizing outcomes and improving quality of life in patients with urticaria. Further research into the mechanisms of action, efficacy, and safety of pharmacological agents for urticaria may lead to advancements in disease management and personalized treatment strategies for this common dermatological condition.

Non-pharmacological Interventions for Urticaria: A Holistic Approach to Management

Urticaria, characterized by the sudden appearance of wheals, angioedema, and pruritus, can significantly impact patients' quality of life. While pharmacological interventions play a crucial role in managing urticaria symptoms, non-pharmacological interventions are also important in reducing symptom severity, preventing exacerbations, and improving overall well-being. This comprehensive review will explore non-pharmacological interventions for urticaria, including trigger avoidance, lifestyle modifications, and stress management techniques, highlighting their importance in holistic disease management.

Non-pharmacological Interventions

Non-pharmacological interventions for urticaria focus on identifying and avoiding triggers, adopting healthy lifestyle habits, and implementing stress management techniques to reduce symptom burden and improve quality of life. These interventions are often used in conjunction with pharmacological therapies to achieve optimal disease control and minimize reliance on medications.

Trigger Avoidance

Identifying and avoiding triggers is a cornerstone of managing urticaria, as exposure to certain allergens, irritants, or environmental factors can precipitate or exacerbate symptoms in susceptible individuals. Common triggers for urticaria include:

- Allergens: Food allergies (e.g., nuts, shellfish, eggs, dairy), airborne allergens (e.g., pollen, pet dander, dust mites), insect stings, and medications (e.g., antibiotics, non-steroidal anti-inflammatory drugs).
- Physical stimuli: Pressure (e.g., tight clothing, sitting for prolonged periods), temperature extremes (e.g., cold, heat), sunlight (e.g., solar urticaria), water (e.g., aquagenic urticaria), and vibration (e.g., vibratory urticaria).
- Emotional stress: Psychological stress, anxiety, and emotional upheaval can trigger or exacerbate urticaria symptoms through neurogenic mechanisms and immune dysregulation.

Patients with urticaria should undergo comprehensive evaluation to identify potential triggers and develop personalized trigger avoidance strategies. This may involve allergen testing, environmental assessments, dietary modifications, and lifestyle changes to minimize exposure to known triggers. Keeping a symptom diary and tracking potential triggers can help patients identify patterns and make informed decisions about trigger avoidance strategies.

Lifestyle Modifications

Adopting healthy lifestyle habits can help improve overall health and well-being in patients with urticaria, potentially reducing symptom severity and frequency. Lifestyle modifications that may benefit patients with urticaria include:

- Diet: Following a balanced diet rich in fruits, vegetables, whole grains, and lean proteins may help support immune function and reduce inflammation. Patients with food allergies or sensitivities should avoid trigger foods and consider working with a registered dietitian to develop personalized meal plans.
- Exercise: Regular physical activity can help reduce stress, improve mood, and enhance overall cardiovascular health. Patients with exercise-induced urticaria should engage in low-impact activities and consider pre-treatment with antihistamines or leukotriene antagonists to prevent symptoms.
- Sleep: Adequate sleep is essential for maintaining immune function, regulating inflammation, and promoting overall health. Patients with urticaria should prioritize good sleep hygiene practices, such as establishing a consistent sleep schedule, creating a relaxing bedtime routine, and optimizing sleep environment.
- Smoking and alcohol: Smoking and excessive alcohol consumption can exacerbate inflammation, weaken immune function, and trigger urticaria symptoms in susceptible individuals. Patients with urticaria should avoid smoking and limit alcohol intake to reduce symptom severity and improve treatment outcomes.
- Skincare: Using gentle, fragrance-free skincare products and avoiding harsh chemicals or irritants can help minimize skin irritation and reduce the risk of triggering urticaria flares. Moisturizing regularly and protecting the skin from environmental stressors can help maintain skin barrier function and prevent dryness or irritation.

Stress Management Techniques

Stress management techniques play a vital role in managing urticaria, as stress and emotional upheaval can exacerbate symptoms through neurogenic mechanisms and immune dysregulation. Patients with urticaria should adopt stress management techniques to reduce symptom severity and improve overall well-being. These techniques may include:

- Relaxation techniques: Practicing relaxation techniques such as deep breathing, progressive muscle relaxation, guided imagery, and meditation can help reduce stress, promote relaxation, and alleviate urticaria symptoms. Patients can incorporate these techniques into their daily routine or use them as needed during times of stress or anxiety.
- Mindfulness-based therapies: Mindfulness-based therapies such as mindfulness-based stress reduction (MBSR) and mindfulness-based cognitive therapy (MBCT) have been shown to reduce stress, improve mood, and enhance overall well-being in patients with chronic conditions, including urticaria. These therapies focus on cultivating present-moment awareness, acceptance, and non-judgmental observation of thoughts and emotions.
- Cognitive-behavioral therapy (CBT): Cognitive-behavioral therapy (CBT) is a psychotherapeutic approach that helps individuals identify and challenge negative thought patterns, develop coping strategies, and modify maladaptive behaviors. CBT can be effective in reducing stress, anxiety, and depression in patients with urticaria, leading to improvements in symptom control and quality of life.
- Support groups: Joining support groups or seeking support from peers, friends, family members, or mental health professionals can provide validation, encouragement, and coping strategies for patients with urticaria. Connecting with others who understand their experiences can help patients feel less isolated and more empowered to manage their condition effectively.

Conclusion

In conclusion, non-pharmacological interventions play a crucial role in managing urticaria, reducing symptom severity, and improving overall well-being in affected individuals. Trigger avoidance strategies, lifestyle modifications, and stress management techniques are essential components of holistic disease management, complementing pharmacological therapies and optimizing treatment outcomes. Healthcare providers should educate patients about the importance of non-pharmacological interventions and empower them to incorporate these strategies into their daily lives to achieve optimal symptom control and improve quality of life. Further research into the effectiveness, feasibility, and long-term benefits of non-pharmacological interventions for urticaria may lead to advancements in disease management and personalized treatment approaches for this common dermatological condition.

Exploring Investigational Therapies and Emerging Treatments for Urticaria

Urticaria, characterized by the sudden appearance of wheals, angioedema, and pruritus, can significantly impact patients' quality of life. While existing pharmacological and non-pharmacological treatments provide relief for many patients, there remains a subset of individuals with refractory or severe disease who may benefit from investigational therapies and emerging treatments. This comprehensive review will explore investigational therapies and emerging treatments for urticaria, highlighting promising approaches that may offer new avenues for disease management and improved patient outcomes.

Investigational Therapies and Emerging Treatments

Advances in understanding the underlying pathophysiology of urticaria have led to the exploration of novel therapeutic targets and treatment modalities aimed at addressing the diverse mechanisms driving the disease. Investigational therapies and emerging treatments for urticaria encompass a wide range of approaches, including biologics, small molecules, immunomodulators, and targeted therapies, each offering unique opportunities for personalized treatment and improved disease control.

Biologics:

Biologic agents targeting specific inflammatory pathways implicated in the pathogenesis of urticaria have shown promise in clinical trials and real-world studies. Omalizumab, a monoclonal antibody targeting IgE, has emerged as a breakthrough treatment for chronic spontaneous urticaria refractory to conventional therapies. By binding to free IgE and preventing its interaction with mast cells and basophils, omalizumab effectively reduces symptom severity, improves quality of life, and provides long-term disease control in many patients.

Other biologics under investigation for the treatment of urticaria include dupilumab, a monoclonal antibody targeting the interleukin-4 receptor alpha subunit, and benralizumab, a monoclonal antibody targeting the interleukin-5 receptor alpha subunit. These agents modulate inflammatory pathways involved in the pathogenesis of urticaria, offering potential alternatives for patients who do not respond to or tolerate conventional therapies.

Small Molecules:

Small molecule inhibitors targeting specific enzymes, receptors, or signaling pathways implicated in urticaria pathophysiology are also under investigation as potential treatment options. Bruton's tyrosine kinase (BTK) inhibitors, such as fenebrutinib and rilzabrutinib, have shown promise in preclinical studies and early-phase clinical trials for the treatment of autoimmune and inflammatory conditions, including chronic spontaneous urticaria. By inhibiting BTK, these agents modulate B-cell signaling, reduce antibody production, and attenuate immune responses, offering a novel approach to managing urticaria.

Other small molecules targeting histamine receptors, leukotriene receptors, or pro-inflammatory cytokines are also being explored for their potential efficacy in urticaria treatment. These agents may offer alternative treatment options for patients who do not respond to or tolerate conventional therapies, providing personalized treatment approaches based on individual disease characteristics and underlying pathophysiology.

Immunomodulators:

Immunomodulatory agents, such as methotrexate, cyclosporine, and mycophenolate mofetil, have traditionally been used off-label in the treatment of severe, refractory urticaria. While effective in some patients, these agents carry the risk of significant adverse effects and may require close monitoring and dose adjustments. Newer immunomodulators with improved safety profiles and targeted mechanisms of action are under investigation for their potential efficacy in urticaria treatment.

Janus kinase (JAK) inhibitors, such as tofacitinib and baricitinib, are oral immunomodulatory agents that target the JAK-STAT signaling pathway, which plays a central role in immune responses and inflammation. These agents modulate cytokine signaling, reduce inflammatory mediators, and attenuate immune dysregulation, offering a novel approach to managing urticaria. Clinical trials evaluating the efficacy and safety of JAK inhibitors in urticaria treatment are underway, with preliminary results showing promising outcomes in some patients.

Targeted Therapies:

Targeted therapies aimed at specific cellular or molecular targets implicated in urticaria pathophysiology offer potential opportunities for personalized treatment and improved disease control. Mast cell stabilizers, such as cromolyn sodium and ketotifen, inhibit mast cell degranulation and release of inflammatory mediators, providing symptomatic relief for some patients with urticaria.

Other targeted therapies under investigation for urticaria treatment include phosphodiesterase-4 (PDE4) inhibitors, neurokinin-1 receptor antagonists, and neurotrophin receptor inhibitors, which modulate various pathways involved in itch sensation, neurogenic inflammation, and mast cell activation. These targeted therapies may offer novel treatment options for patients with refractory or severe urticaria unresponsive to conventional therapies, providing opportunities for personalized treatment approaches based on individual disease characteristics and underlying pathophysiology.

Conclusion:

In conclusion, investigational therapies and emerging treatments for urticaria offer promising opportunities for improved disease management and patient outcomes. Biologics, small molecules, immunomodulators, and targeted therapies targeting specific inflammatory pathways or cellular/molecular targets implicated in urticaria pathophysiology may provide alternative treatment options for patients who do not respond to or tolerate conventional therapies. Further research into the efficacy, safety, and long-term benefits of these investigational therapies is needed to establish their role in urticaria treatment and inform personalized treatment approaches for this common dermatological condition. Collaborative efforts between researchers, healthcare providers, and industry partners are essential for advancing our understanding of urticaria pathophysiology and developing innovative therapies to address the unmet needs of patients with refractory or severe disease.

Empowering Patients Through Education and Counseling: Enhancing Understanding and Management of Urticaria

Patient education and counseling play a pivotal role in the comprehensive management of urticaria, a condition characterized by the sudden onset of wheals, angioedema, and pruritus. By providing patients with accurate information about the disease, its triggers, treatment options, and self-management strategies, healthcare providers can empower individuals to take an active role in managing their condition and improving their quality of life. This comprehensive review will explore the importance of patient education and counseling in urticaria management, highlighting key components and strategies for enhancing patient understanding and engagement.

Patient Education and Counseling

Understanding Urticaria:

Effective patient education begins with providing individuals with a clear understanding of urticaria, including its symptoms, triggers, underlying mechanisms, and treatment options. Patients should be informed that urticaria is a common dermatological condition characterized by the sudden appearance of wheals (hives) and/or angioedema (swelling) on the skin, often accompanied by intense itching. They should understand that urticaria can be triggered by various factors, including allergens, physical stimuli, emotional stress, and underlying medical conditions, and that the exact cause may be difficult to identify in some cases.

Treatment Options:

Patients should be educated about the different treatment options available for urticaria, including pharmacological therapies, non-pharmacological interventions, and lifestyle modifications. Healthcare providers should discuss the benefits and potential risks of each treatment option, as well as factors to consider when making treatment decisions, such as disease severity, treatment goals, comorbidities, and individual preferences. Patients should be encouraged to actively participate in treatment decision-making and to communicate openly with their healthcare providers about their concerns, preferences, and treatment expectations.

Self-Management Strategies:

In addition to pharmacological therapies, patients with urticaria can benefit from adopting self-management strategies to reduce symptom severity, prevent exacerbations, and improve overall well-being. Healthcare providers should educate patients about trigger avoidance techniques, lifestyle modifications, and stress management techniques that can help minimize the impact of urticaria on daily life. Patients should be encouraged to keep a symptom diary to track potential triggers and patterns of symptom exacerbation, and to seek medical attention if they experience severe or persistent symptoms despite self-management efforts.

Medication Adherence:

Patient education should also focus on promoting medication adherence and ensuring that patients understand how to use their prescribed medications safely and effectively. Healthcare providers should provide clear instructions on medication dosing, administration, and potential side effects, as well as strategies for managing medication-related issues such as drug interactions, adverse reactions, and treatment non-compliance. Patients should be encouraged to ask questions, seek clarification, and voice any concerns or barriers to medication adherence, and healthcare providers should address these concerns in a non-judgmental and supportive manner.

Psychosocial Impact:

Urticaria can have a significant psychosocial impact on patients, affecting their emotional well-being, social interactions, and overall quality of life. Healthcare providers should acknowledge the psychosocial impact of urticaria and provide patients with emotional support, reassurance, and coping strategies to help them manage the emotional aspects of living with a chronic skin condition. Patients should be encouraged to seek support from friends, family members, support groups, or mental health professionals as needed, and healthcare providers should facilitate access to appropriate resources and referrals.

Shared Decision-Making:

Shared decision-making is an essential component of patient-centered care, empowering patients to actively participate in their healthcare decisions and collaborate with their healthcare providers to achieve mutually agreed-upon treatment goals. Healthcare providers should engage patients in shared decision-making by providing them with accurate information, discussing treatment options, eliciting patient preferences and values, and considering patient preferences and priorities when making treatment decisions. Patients should be encouraged to ask questions, express their concerns and preferences, and actively participate in the decision-making process, ensuring that their individual needs and preferences are respected and addressed.

Counseling and Support:

Counseling and support services can play a valuable role in helping patients cope with the challenges of living with urticaria and develop effective coping strategies to manage their condition. Healthcare providers should assess patients' psychosocial needs and provide counseling, emotional support, and practical guidance to help patients navigate the emotional and practical aspects of living with urticaria. Patients should be encouraged to seek counseling or support from mental health professionals, support groups, or other resources as needed, and healthcare providers should facilitate access to these services and provide ongoing support and encouragement.

Conclusion:

In conclusion, patient education and counseling are essential components of urticaria management, empowering patients to take an active role in managing their condition and improving their quality of life. By providing patients with accurate information about the disease, its triggers, treatment options, and self-management strategies, healthcare providers can help patients make informed decisions about their care, enhance treatment adherence, and optimize treatment outcomes. Effective patient education and counseling require a collaborative, patient-centered approach that acknowledges patients' individual needs, preferences, and values, and supports their active participation in the healthcare decision-making process. By prioritizing patient education and counseling, healthcare providers can empower patients to effectively manage their urticaria and achieve better health outcomes.

CHAPTER 7: IMPACT ON QUALITY OF LIFE AND PSYCHOSOCIAL CONSIDERATIONS

Understanding the Psychological Impact of Chronic Hives

Chronic hives, also known as chronic idiopathic urticaria, is a dermatological condition characterized by the recurrent appearance of wheals, angioedema, and itching lasting for more than six weeks. While the physical symptoms of chronic hives are often the focus of medical attention, it is essential to recognize and address the significant psychological impact that this condition can have on affected individuals. This comprehensive review will explore the psychological impact of chronic hives, including its effects on mental health, emotional well-being, social interactions, and quality of life.

Psychological Impact of Chronic Hives

Emotional Distress:

Living with chronic hives can be emotionally distressing, as patients grapple with the uncertainty of when symptoms will occur, the unpredictability of symptom severity, and the constant discomfort and itching associated with the condition. The chronic nature of hives can lead to feelings of frustration, anxiety, and depression, as patients struggle to cope with the physical symptoms and the impact they have on their daily lives. Many patients report feeling overwhelmed by the constant need to manage their symptoms, leading to feelings of helplessness and despair.

Impact on Mental Health:

Chronic hives can have a significant impact on mental health, contributing to the development or exacerbation of mental health conditions such as anxiety disorders, depression, and obsessive-compulsive disorder (OCD). The persistent itching and discomfort associated with hives can disrupt sleep patterns, impair concentration and cognitive function, and interfere with daily activities, leading to feelings of fatigue, irritability, and impaired social functioning. Patients may experience heightened levels of stress and psychological distress, which can further exacerbate their hives symptoms in a vicious cycle.

Social Isolation:

The visible nature of hives lesions and the associated stigma surrounding skin conditions can lead to social isolation and withdrawal from social activities. Patients may feel self-conscious about their appearance and reluctant to engage in social interactions or participate in activities that expose their skin, such as swimming, sports, or wearing revealing clothing. Social isolation can exacerbate feelings of loneliness, low self-esteem, and poor body image, further impacting patients' mental health and overall quality of life.

Impact on Quality of Life:

Chronic hives can have a profound impact on the quality of life of affected individuals, impairing their ability to perform daily activities, pursue hobbies and interests, and maintain relationships with family and friends. The physical discomfort and psychological distress associated with hives can diminish patients' overall sense of well-being and satisfaction with life, leading to decreased productivity, impaired social functioning, and reduced participation in meaningful activities. Patients may struggle to cope with the emotional and practical challenges of living with a chronic skin condition, which can negatively impact their quality of life and overall health outcomes.

Coping Strategies:

Despite the challenges posed by chronic hives, many patients develop effective coping strategies to manage their symptoms and improve their psychological well-being. These coping strategies may include seeking social support from friends, family members, or support groups, engaging in stress-reduction techniques such as mindfulness meditation or relaxation exercises, and maintaining a positive outlook and resilience in the face of adversity. Psychotherapy and counseling can also be valuable tools for patients struggling to cope with the emotional impact of chronic hives, providing them with the support, guidance, and coping skills needed to navigate the challenges of living with a chronic skin condition.

Conclusion:

In conclusion, chronic hives can have a significant psychological impact on affected individuals, contributing to emotional distress, mental health issues, social isolation, and impaired quality of life. It is essential for healthcare providers to recognize and address the psychological aspects of chronic hives, as well as to provide patients with comprehensive care that addresses both the physical and emotional aspects of their condition. By implementing multidisciplinary approaches that incorporate psychosocial support, counseling, and education, healthcare providers can help patients effectively manage their symptoms, improve their psychological well-being, and enhance their overall quality of life. Additionally, raising awareness about the psychological impact of chronic hives among healthcare providers, patients, and the general public can help reduce stigma, increase understanding, and promote empathy and support for individuals living with this challenging condition.

Effective Coping Strategies for Managing Chronic Hives

Living with chronic hives, a condition characterized by recurrent outbreaks of wheals, itching, and swelling, can pose significant challenges for affected individuals. Coping with the physical symptoms, emotional distress, and lifestyle disruptions associated with chronic hives requires the implementation of effective coping strategies. This section explores various coping strategies that can help individuals manage the impact of chronic hives on their daily lives and overall well-being.

Coping Strategies

1. Education and Understanding:

- Educate yourself about chronic hives, including its triggers, symptoms, and treatment options. Understanding your condition can help you feel more empowered and in control of your health.

2. Stress Management Techniques:

- Practice stress management techniques such as deep breathing, meditation, yoga, or progressive muscle relaxation to reduce stress levels and promote relaxation. Stress can exacerbate hives symptoms, so finding ways to manage stress effectively is essential.

3. Trigger Identification and Avoidance:

- Identify and avoid triggers that exacerbate your hives symptoms, such as certain foods, environmental allergens, or emotional stressors. Keeping a symptom diary can help you track potential triggers and make informed decisions about lifestyle modifications.

4. Skincare and Symptom Management:

- Follow a gentle skincare routine to soothe irritated skin and minimize itching. Use fragrance-free, hypoallergenic skincare products, and moisturize regularly to maintain skin hydration and integrity. Apply cool compresses or take lukewarm baths to alleviate itching during flare-ups.

5. Medication Adherence:

- Adhere to your prescribed medication regimen as directed by your healthcare provider. Take medications consistently and as prescribed to maintain symptom control and prevent flare-ups. Communicate any concerns or side effects with your healthcare provider promptly.

6. Support Networks:

- Seek support from friends, family members, or support groups who understand and empathize with your condition. Sharing your experiences with others who are going through similar challenges can provide validation, encouragement, and a sense of belonging.

7. Positive Coping Strategies:

- Focus on activities and hobbies that bring you joy, fulfillment, and a sense of accomplishment. Engage in activities that distract you from hives symptoms and promote relaxation and well-being, such as spending time outdoors, practicing creative arts, or connecting with loved ones.

8. Cognitive-Behavioral Techniques:

- Practice cognitive-behavioral techniques to challenge negative thought patterns and develop adaptive coping strategies. Replace catastrophic thinking with more realistic and positive perspectives, and learn to reframe setbacks as opportunities for growth and resilience.

9. Professional Support:

- Consider seeking professional support from a therapist, counselor, or psychologist who specializes in chronic illness or dermatological conditions. Therapy can provide you with tools and strategies to cope effectively with the emotional challenges of living with chronic hives and improve your overall quality of life.

10. Self-Compassion:

- Be kind to yourself and practice self-compassion as you navigate the challenges of living with chronic hives. Acknowledge your strengths, accomplishments, and resilience in managing your condition, and treat yourself with the same compassion and understanding you would offer to a loved one facing similar challenges.

Conclusion:

Implementing effective coping strategies is essential for managing the physical symptoms, emotional distress, and lifestyle disruptions associated with chronic hives. By adopting proactive measures to reduce stress, identify triggers, adhere to medication regimens, seek support from others, and engage in positive coping activities, individuals with chronic hives can improve their quality of life and enhance their overall well-being. It is essential to experiment with various coping strategies to determine what works best for you and to seek professional support when needed. With the right support, resources, and coping skills, individuals can effectively manage the challenges of living with chronic hives and lead fulfilling and meaningful lives.

Building Support Networks and Accessing Resources for Chronic Hives

Living with chronic hives, characterized by recurrent episodes of wheals, itching, and swelling, can be challenging and isolating. However, having access to supportive networks and resources can greatly improve the ability of individuals to cope with the physical and emotional aspects of the condition. This section explores the importance of support networks and provides guidance on accessing relevant resources for individuals affected by chronic hives.

Support Networks and Resources

1. Online Support Groups:

- Join online support groups and forums specifically for individuals living with chronic hives. These platforms provide opportunities to connect with others who understand your experiences, share coping strategies, and offer mutual support and encouragement.

2. Patient Advocacy Organizations:

- Explore patient advocacy organizations dedicated to raising awareness about chronic hives and providing support and resources for affected individuals. These organizations often offer educational materials, online forums, support groups, and advocacy initiatives to empower patients and caregivers.

3. Healthcare Providers:

- Build a strong relationship with your healthcare providers, including dermatologists, allergists, and primary care physicians. They can offer guidance, support, and treatment options tailored to your specific needs and preferences.

4. Mental Health Professionals:

- Consider seeking support from mental health professionals, such as therapists, counselors, or psychologists, who specialize in chronic illness or dermatological conditions. Therapy can provide you with tools and strategies to cope effectively with the emotional challenges of living with chronic hives.

5. Educational Resources:

- Educate yourself about chronic hives by accessing reliable educational resources, such as websites, books, and pamphlets provided by reputable healthcare organizations and patient advocacy groups. Understanding your condition can help you make informed decisions about treatment and self-management.

6. Social Support:

- Lean on friends, family members, and loved ones for emotional support and practical assistance. Communicate openly about your experiences with chronic hives and let them know how they can best support you during flare-ups and difficult times.

7. Lifestyle Resources:

- Explore lifestyle resources and self-help materials focused on managing chronic hives symptoms and improving overall well-being. These resources may include tips on skincare, stress management techniques, dietary recommendations, and strategies for enhancing quality of life.

8. Dermatological Clinics and Centers:

- Seek out specialized dermatological clinics and centers that focus on the diagnosis and management of chronic hives. These facilities may offer comprehensive care, access to cutting-edge treatments, and support services tailored to the needs of individuals with chronic skin conditions.

9. Educational Workshops and Webinars:

- Attend educational workshops, webinars, and conferences focused on chronic hives and related dermatological conditions. These events provide opportunities to learn from experts, connect with peers, and stay informed about the latest advancements in research and treatment.

10. Government and Community Resources:

- Explore government and community resources available to individuals with chronic hives, such as public health agencies, social services, and community organizations. These resources may offer financial assistance, social support programs, and access to healthcare services for those in need.

Conclusion:

Support networks and resources play a vital role in helping individuals affected by chronic hives cope with the challenges of living with the condition. By accessing online support groups, patient advocacy organizations, healthcare providers, mental health professionals, educational resources, and community resources, individuals can find the information, support, and guidance they need to navigate their journey with chronic hives effectively. It is essential to reach out for help when needed and to build a strong support network of friends, family, and healthcare providers who can offer encouragement, empathy, and practical assistance along the way. With the right support and resources, individuals with chronic hives can enhance their quality of life and achieve greater well-being.

CHAPTER 8: INTEGRATIVE APPROACHES AND HOLISTIC HEALTH

Exploring Dietary Considerations and Supplements for Chronic Hives Management

Dietary considerations and the use of supplements have been areas of interest for individuals living with chronic hives, seeking additional strategies to manage their symptoms. While the role of diet in the development and exacerbation of chronic hives is not fully understood, certain dietary factors and supplements have been suggested to influence symptom severity and frequency. This section delves into dietary considerations and supplements that individuals with chronic hives may explore as adjunctive measures to their overall management plan.

Dietary Considerations and Supplements

1. Potential Dietary Triggers:

- Some individuals with chronic hives may find that certain foods trigger or exacerbate their symptoms.

Common dietary triggers include shellfish, nuts, eggs, dairy products, food additives (such as sulfites and artificial preservatives), and histamine-rich foods (such as fermented foods and aged cheeses). Keeping a food diary and tracking symptoms can help identify potential dietary triggers, allowing individuals to make informed decisions about their diet.

2. Elimination Diet:

- An elimination diet involves temporarily removing potential dietary triggers from the diet and gradually reintroducing them one at a time to assess their impact on symptoms. This approach can help identify specific foods that may exacerbate hives symptoms in some individuals. It is essential to work with a healthcare provider or registered dietitian when undertaking an elimination diet to ensure nutritional adequacy and avoid unintended consequences.

3. Anti-Inflammatory Diet:

- Adopting an anti-inflammatory diet rich in fruits, vegetables, whole grains, healthy fats (such as omega-3 fatty acids found in fatty fish, flaxseeds, and walnuts), and lean proteins may help reduce inflammation and support overall health. Some individuals with chronic hives may find that following an anti-inflammatory diet helps alleviate symptoms and improves their quality of life.

4. Supplements:

- Certain supplements have been suggested to have potential benefits for individuals with chronic hives. These include:
  - **Quercetin:** Quercetin is a flavonoid found in fruits, vegetables, and supplements. It has anti-inflammatory and antioxidant properties and may help stabilize mast cells, reducing histamine release

and alleviating hives symptoms.

- **Vitamin D:** Vitamin D plays a role in immune regulation and may have anti-inflammatory effects. Some studies suggest that vitamin D supplementation may help reduce the frequency and severity of hives outbreaks in individuals with low vitamin D levels.
- **Omega-3 Fatty Acids:** Omega-3 fatty acids found in fish oil supplements have anti-inflammatory properties and may help modulate immune function. While evidence supporting their use in chronic hives is limited, some individuals may find omega-3 supplementation beneficial.
- **Probiotics:** Probiotics are beneficial bacteria that may help support gut health and immune function. Some research suggests that certain probiotic strains may have anti-inflammatory effects and could potentially benefit individuals with chronic hives by modulating immune responses.

5. Herbal Remedies:

- Certain herbal remedies, such as stinging nettle (Urtica dioica), butterbur (Petasites hybridus), and licorice root (Glycyrrhiza glabra), have been traditionally used for their anti-inflammatory and antihistamine properties. While limited scientific evidence supports their efficacy in chronic hives, some individuals may find herbal remedies helpful as adjunctive measures to their overall management plan.

6. Individualized Approach:

- It is essential to take an individualized approach to dietary considerations and supplement use in chronic hives management. What works for one person may not work for another, and some dietary interventions or supplements may interact with medications or exacerbate underlying health conditions. Consulting with a healthcare provider or registered dietitian can help individuals develop a personalized approach to dietary management and supplement use that is safe, effective, and tailored to their specific needs and preferences.

Conclusion:

Dietary considerations and supplements represent additional strategies that individuals with chronic hives may explore as part of their overall management plan. While the role of diet in chronic hives is not fully understood, some individuals may find that certain dietary modifications or supplements help alleviate symptoms and improve their quality of life. It is essential to approach dietary considerations and supplement use with caution, seeking guidance from healthcare providers or registered dietitians to ensure safety, efficacy, and individualized care. With a personalized approach to dietary management and supplement use, individuals with chronic hives can optimize their symptom control and enhance their overall well-being.

Exploring Acupuncture and Traditional Chinese Medicine for Chronic Hives Management

Acupuncture and Traditional Chinese Medicine (TCM) have been utilized for centuries to treat a wide range of health conditions, including chronic hives. While the mechanisms of action and efficacy of these modalities in the management of chronic hives are not fully understood, some individuals find relief from their symptoms through acupuncture and TCM interventions. This section delves into the principles of acupuncture and TCM and explores their potential role in the management of chronic hives.

Acupuncture and Traditional Chinese Medicine

1. Principles of Acupuncture:

- Acupuncture is a key component of Traditional Chinese Medicine (TCM) and involves the insertion of thin needles into specific points on the body to stimulate energy flow, or Qi, along meridians or energy pathways. According to TCM theory, disruptions in Qi flow can lead to imbalances and manifest as various health conditions, including chronic hives. Acupuncture aims to restore balance and promote healing by unblocking energy channels and regulating the flow of Qi.

2. Acupuncture for Chronic Hives:

- Some individuals with chronic hives may seek acupuncture as an alternative or complementary treatment to conventional therapies. Acupuncture may be used alone or in conjunction with other TCM modalities, such as herbal medicine, dietary therapy, and lifestyle modifications. Acupuncture points selected for the treatment of chronic hives may target areas associated with immune regulation, inflammation, and stress response.

3. Potential Mechanisms of Action:

- The mechanisms by which acupuncture exerts its effects in chronic hives are not fully understood and may involve multiple pathways. Some proposed mechanisms include:
  - Modulation of immune responses: Acupuncture may modulate immune function, including the release of inflammatory mediators and the activity of immune cells involved in the pathogenesis of chronic hives.
  - Regulation of neuroendocrine pathways: Acupuncture may influence neuroendocrine pathways involved in stress response and

inflammation, helping to reduce stress levels and mitigate the impact of psychological factors on hives symptoms.

- Promotion of relaxation and stress reduction: Acupuncture may stimulate the release of endorphins and other neurotransmitters associated with relaxation and stress reduction, providing symptomatic relief for individuals with chronic hives.

4. Clinical Evidence and Research:

- Clinical evidence supporting the use of acupuncture for chronic hives is limited and mixed, with some studies reporting positive outcomes and others showing no significant benefits compared to sham acupuncture or conventional therapies. More research is needed to better understand the efficacy, safety, and optimal protocols for acupuncture in chronic hives management.

5. Considerations and Precautions:

- Individuals considering acupuncture for chronic hives should consult with a qualified acupuncturist or healthcare provider experienced in TCM. It is essential to discuss treatment goals, expectations, and any underlying health conditions or medications that may affect treatment outcomes. Acupuncture is generally considered safe when performed by trained practitioners using sterile needles and appropriate techniques. However, individuals with bleeding disorders, immune disorders, or other medical conditions should exercise caution and seek guidance from their healthcare provider.

6. Integrative Approach:

- Acupuncture and TCM can be integrated into a comprehensive treatment plan for chronic hives, alongside conventional therapies, lifestyle modifications, and other complementary modalities. An integrative approach allows for personalized care tailored to the individual needs and preferences of each patient, maximizing symptom control and overall well-being.

Conclusion:

Acupuncture and Traditional Chinese Medicine offer potential avenues for individuals with chronic hives to explore as part of their overall management plan. While the mechanisms of action and clinical evidence supporting their use in chronic hives are still evolving, some individuals may find relief from their symptoms through acupuncture and TCM interventions. It is essential to approach acupuncture and TCM with an open mind, seek guidance from qualified practitioners, and integrate these modalities into a comprehensive treatment plan that addresses the multifaceted nature of chronic hives. With careful consideration and personalized care, individuals with chronic hives can optimize their symptom control and enhance their overall quality of life.

Exploring Herbal Remedies and Naturopathic Approaches for Chronic Hives Management

Herbal remedies and naturopathic approaches have been utilized for centuries in various traditional healing systems to address a wide range of health conditions, including chronic hives. While the scientific evidence supporting the efficacy of these interventions in the management of chronic hives is limited, some individuals find relief from their symptoms through the use of herbal remedies and naturopathic approaches. This section delves into the principles of herbal medicine and naturopathy and explores their potential role in the management of chronic hives.

Herbal Remedies and Naturopathic Approaches

1. Principles of Herbal Medicine:

- Herbal medicine involves the use of plant-based remedies, including herbs, roots, flowers, and bark, to promote health and alleviate symptoms of illness. Herbal remedies are often prepared as teas, tinctures, capsules, or topical preparations and may contain a combination of active constituents with potential therapeutic effects.

2. Herbal Remedies for Chronic Hives:

- Several herbs and botanical extracts have been traditionally used in the management of skin conditions, including chronic hives. Common herbal remedies for chronic hives include:
    - **Stinging Nettle (Urtica dioica):** Stinging nettle has anti-inflammatory properties and may help reduce itching and inflammation associated with hives.
    - **Butterbur (Petasites hybridus):** Butterbur has anti-inflammatory and antihistamine properties and may help alleviate hives symptoms.
    - **Licorice Root (Glycyrrhiza glabra):** Licorice root has anti-inflammatory and immune-modulating properties and may help reduce inflammation and immune system activation in chronic hives.
    - **Turmeric (Curcuma longa):** Turmeric contains curcumin, a compound with anti-inflammatory and antioxidant properties that may help alleviate inflammation and itching in chronic hives.

3. Naturopathic Approaches:

- Naturopathic medicine emphasizes the use of natural therapies, lifestyle modifications, and holistic approaches to promote health and treat illness. Naturopathic approaches for chronic hives may include:

- **Dietary Modifications:** Identifying and eliminating potential dietary triggers, such as food allergens or histamine-rich foods, may help reduce hives symptoms. Some individuals may benefit from adopting an anti-inflammatory diet rich in fruits, vegetables, and omega-3 fatty acids to support overall health and immune function.

- **Lifestyle Modifications:** Stress management techniques, such as meditation, yoga, and deep breathing exercises, may help reduce stress levels and minimize the impact of psychological factors on hives symptoms. Avoiding environmental triggers, such as extreme temperatures, tight clothing, and harsh chemicals, may also help prevent flare-ups.

- **Supplements:** Certain supplements, such as quercetin, vitamin D, omega-3 fatty acids, and probiotics, have been suggested to have potential benefits for individuals with chronic hives. However, evidence supporting their use in hives management is limited, and individuals should exercise caution and consult with a healthcare provider before starting any new supplement regimen.

4. Clinical Evidence and Research:

- The scientific evidence supporting the efficacy of herbal remedies and naturopathic approaches in the management of chronic hives is limited and inconclusive. While some studies suggest potential benefits for certain herbs and natural therapies, more research is needed to establish their safety, efficacy, and optimal use in hives management.

5. Safety and Precautions:

- It is essential to approach herbal remedies and naturopathic approaches with caution and consult with a qualified healthcare provider before starting any new treatment regimen. Some herbs may interact with medications or exacerbate underlying health conditions, and individual responses to herbal remedies can vary. Pregnant or breastfeeding individuals, as well as children and individuals with certain medical conditions, should exercise particular caution and seek guidance from a healthcare provider.

Conclusion:

Herbal remedies and naturopathic approaches offer potential avenues for individuals with chronic hives to explore as part of their overall management plan. While the scientific evidence supporting their efficacy in hives management is limited, some individuals may find relief from their symptoms through the use of herbal remedies and naturopathic interventions. It is essential to approach these modalities with an open mind, seek guidance from qualified practitioners, and integrate them into a comprehensive treatment plan that addresses the multifaceted nature of chronic hives. With careful consideration and personalized care, individuals with chronic hives can optimize their symptom control and enhance their overall quality of life.

Exploring Mind-Body Practices for Chronic Hives Management

Mind-body practices, such as yoga, meditation, and mindfulness, have gained recognition for their potential to promote relaxation, reduce stress, and enhance overall well-being. For individuals living with chronic hives, incorporating mind-body practices into their management plan may offer additional strategies for coping with the physical and emotional challenges associated with the condition. This section explores the principles of mind-body practices and their potential role in the management of chronic hives.

Mind-Body Practices

1. Yoga:

- Yoga is a mind-body practice that combines physical postures, breathing techniques, and meditation to promote relaxation, flexibility, and mindfulness. For individuals with chronic hives, practicing yoga may help reduce stress levels, improve immune function, and alleviate inflammation, potentially leading to a reduction in hives symptoms. Certain yoga poses, such as forward bends and twists, may also stimulate circulation and lymphatic drainage, supporting skin health and reducing inflammation.

2. Meditation:

- Meditation involves the practice of focusing attention and cultivating awareness of the present moment, often through techniques such as mindfulness meditation, guided imagery, or loving-kindness meditation. Regular meditation practice has been associated with reduced stress levels, improved mood, and enhanced immune function, all of which may benefit individuals with chronic hives. By promoting relaxation and reducing psychological distress, meditation may help mitigate the impact of stress on hives symptoms and improve overall well-being.

3. Mindfulness:

- Mindfulness involves paying attention to thoughts, feelings, and sensations in the present moment with an attitude of openness and non-judgment. Mindfulness practices, such as mindful breathing, body scans, and mindful eating, can help individuals with chronic hives cultivate greater awareness of their body's responses and develop more adaptive coping strategies for managing stress and discomfort. By fostering a sense of acceptance and equanimity, mindfulness may reduce the intensity of hives symptoms and improve psychological resilience.

4. Relaxation Techniques:

- Various relaxation techniques, such as progressive muscle relaxation, deep breathing exercises, and guided imagery, can help induce a state of relaxation and counteract the physiological effects of stress on the body. Incorporating these relaxation techniques into daily life can help individuals with chronic hives manage stress more effectively, reduce muscle tension, and promote a sense of calm and well-being.

5. Biofeedback:

- Biofeedback is a mind-body technique that involves using electronic monitoring devices to provide real-time feedback on physiological processes, such as heart rate variability, muscle tension, and skin temperature. By learning to control these physiological responses through relaxation techniques and mental imagery, individuals with chronic hives can potentially reduce the frequency and severity of hives symptoms and improve their overall quality of life.

6. Tai Chi and Qigong:

- Tai Chi and Qigong are mind-body practices originating from traditional Chinese martial arts that involve slow, gentle movements, coordinated breathing, and meditation. These practices promote balance, flexibility, and energy flow, and may help reduce stress levels, improve immune function, and enhance overall well-being in individuals with chronic hives.

Conclusion:

Mind-body practices offer promising avenues for individuals with chronic hives to explore as part of their overall management plan. By incorporating practices such as yoga, meditation, mindfulness, relaxation techniques, biofeedback, and Tai Chi/Qigong into their daily routine, individuals can cultivate greater resilience, reduce stress levels, and improve their ability to cope with the physical and emotional challenges of living with chronic hives. It is essential to approach mind-body practices with an open mind, engage in regular practice, and seek guidance from qualified instructors or healthcare providers to ensure safe and effective implementation. With consistent practice and commitment, individuals with chronic hives can enhance their symptom control and achieve greater well-being.

CHAPTER 9: FUTURE DIRECTIONS IN CHRONIC HIVES RESEARCH

Exploring Advances in Immunotherapy for Chronic Hives

Immunotherapy, which aims to modulate the immune system's response, has emerged as a promising approach for the management of chronic hives. Recent advances in immunotherapy have led to the development of targeted therapies that specifically address underlying immune dysregulation associated with chronic hives. This section explores the latest advances in immunotherapy and their potential implications for the treatment of chronic hives.

Advances in Immunotherapy

1. Omalizumab (Xolair):

- Omalizumab is a monoclonal antibody that targets immunoglobulin E (IgE), a key mediator of allergic responses. While initially approved for the treatment of allergic asthma and chronic idiopathic urticaria

(CIU), omalizumab has shown promising results in the management of chronic hives refractory to conventional therapies. By binding to circulating IgE antibodies and preventing their interaction with mast cells and basophils, omalizumab helps reduce the release of histamine and other inflammatory mediators, thereby alleviating hives symptoms.

2. Anti-IL-5 and Anti-IL-4/IL-13 Therapies:

- Interleukin-5 (IL-5) and interleukin-4 (IL-4)/interleukin-13 (IL-13) are cytokines involved in the regulation of eosinophilic inflammation and type 2 immune responses, which may play a role in the pathogenesis of chronic hives. Several biologic therapies targeting IL-5 (e.g., mepolizumab, reslizumab) and IL-4/IL-13 (e.g., dupilumab) have shown efficacy in the treatment of eosinophilic disorders and atopic dermatitis, respectively. While their role in chronic hives is still being investigated, these therapies represent promising avenues for targeted immunomodulation in refractory cases.

3. Janus Kinase (JAK) Inhibitors:

- Janus kinase (JAK) inhibitors are small molecule drugs that inhibit the activity of JAK enzymes involved in cytokine signaling pathways. Emerging evidence suggests that dysregulation of JAK/STAT signaling may contribute to the pathogenesis of chronic hives. Tofacitinib, a JAK inhibitor, has demonstrated efficacy in the treatment of autoimmune and inflammatory conditions and may hold potential for the management of chronic hives. Clinical trials evaluating the safety and efficacy of JAK inhibitors in chronic hives are currently underway.

4. Autologous Serum Therapy:

- Autologous serum therapy involves the injection of a

patient's own serum, which has been processed to remove immune complexes and other potentially pathogenic factors, back into the patient's skin. While the mechanism of action is not fully understood, autologous serum therapy has shown promising results in the treatment of refractory chronic hives. By exposing the immune system to small amounts of autologous serum, this therapy may help desensitize patients to their own autoantibodies and modulate aberrant immune responses.

5. Allergen-Specific Immunotherapy:

- Allergen-specific immunotherapy (AIT), commonly known as allergy shots, involves the gradual administration of increasing doses of allergen extracts to induce immune tolerance and reduce allergic symptoms. While traditionally used for the treatment of allergic rhinitis and asthma, AIT has shown potential as a treatment option for chronic hives associated with specific allergens. By targeting the underlying allergic triggers, AIT may help alleviate hives symptoms and reduce the need for symptomatic medications.

6. Personalized and Precision Medicine Approaches:

- Advances in personalized and precision medicine have paved the way for tailored treatment approaches based on individual patient characteristics, including immune profiles, genetic factors, and environmental triggers. By identifying specific immune pathways and biomarkers associated with chronic hives, clinicians can develop targeted immunotherapy strategies that address the underlying pathophysiology of the condition and optimize treatment outcomes for each patient.

Conclusion:

Advances in immunotherapy hold great promise for the

management of chronic hives, offering targeted approaches that address underlying immune dysregulation and provide relief for patients with refractory symptoms. From monoclonal antibodies targeting IgE and cytokines to small molecule inhibitors and innovative therapies like autologous serum therapy and allergen-specific immunotherapy, the landscape of immunotherapy for chronic hives is rapidly evolving. With ongoing research and clinical trials, the future holds exciting possibilities for personalized and precision medicine approaches that enhance the effectiveness and safety of immunotherapy for chronic hives.

Exploring Precision Medicine Approaches for Chronic Hives

Precision medicine, also known as personalized medicine, aims to tailor medical treatment to the individual characteristics of each patient, including genetic makeup, biomarkers, and environmental factors. In the context of chronic hives, precision medicine approaches offer the potential to identify specific immune pathways, allergic triggers, and genetic predispositions that contribute to the condition's pathogenesis. This section delves into precision medicine approaches for chronic hives and their implications for personalized treatment strategies.

Precision Medicine Approaches

1. Immune Profiling:

- Immune profiling involves the analysis of immune cells, cytokines, and other immune markers to characterize the immune response in individuals with chronic hives. By identifying patterns of immune dysregulation and inflammatory mediators associated with the condition, immune profiling can help guide targeted treatment approaches that address underlying pathophysiological mechanisms.

2. Genetic Testing:

- Genetic testing allows for the identification of genetic variants and polymorphisms that may influence an individual's susceptibility to chronic hives and their response to treatment. Genome-wide association studies (GWAS) and targeted genetic sequencing can reveal genetic factors associated with the condition, such as variations in genes encoding for immunoglobulins, cytokines, and immune receptors. Understanding the genetic basis of chronic hives can inform personalized treatment strategies and help identify individuals at higher risk for severe or refractory disease.

3. Biomarker Analysis:

- Biomarker analysis involves the identification of molecular markers in blood, serum, or tissue samples that correlate with disease activity, severity, or treatment response. Biomarkers associated with chronic hives may include serum levels of IgE, histamine, cytokines, and autoantibodies. By monitoring changes in biomarker expression over time, clinicians can assess treatment efficacy, predict disease progression, and tailor therapeutic interventions to individual patient needs.

4. Environmental Triggers Assessment:

- Precision medicine approaches for chronic hives also encompass the identification and avoidance of environmental triggers that exacerbate symptoms in susceptible individuals. Comprehensive environmental assessments, including allergen testing, environmental exposure history, and lifestyle factors, can help pinpoint specific triggers, such as allergens, pollutants, stressors, and dietary factors. By minimizing exposure to triggers and modifying lifestyle habits, individuals can reduce the frequency and severity of hives outbreaks and optimize treatment outcomes.

5. Personalized Treatment Plans:

- Based on the findings from immune profiling, genetic testing, biomarker analysis, and environmental assessments, clinicians can develop personalized treatment plans tailored to the unique needs and characteristics of each patient. Precision medicine approaches may involve a combination of targeted immunotherapy, pharmacological interventions, lifestyle modifications, and patient education strategies aimed at addressing the underlying mechanisms driving chronic hives and optimizing symptom control.

6. Integration of Digital Health Technologies:

- Digital health technologies, such as wearable devices, smartphone applications, and telemedicine platforms, play a growing role in facilitating precision medicine approaches for chronic hives. These technologies enable remote monitoring of symptoms, medication adherence, and treatment responses, allowing for real-time adjustments to treatment plans and enhanced patient-provider communication. By integrating digital health tools into precision medicine initiatives, healthcare providers can deliver personalized care and support to individuals with chronic hives, improving outcomes and patient satisfaction.

Conclusion:

Precision medicine approaches offer a promising paradigm shift in the management of chronic hives, allowing for personalized treatment strategies that address the underlying immune dysregulation, genetic factors, and environmental triggers contributing to the condition. By leveraging immune profiling, genetic testing, biomarker analysis, environmental assessments, and digital health technologies, clinicians can develop tailored treatment plans that optimize symptom control and improve quality of life for individuals with chronic hives. As research continues to advance in the field of precision medicine, the future holds exciting possibilities for personalized, targeted therapies that transform the management of chronic hives and enhance patient outcomes.

Exploring Biomarkers for Disease Monitoring in Chronic Hives

Biomarkers play a crucial role in disease monitoring by providing objective measures of disease activity, severity, and treatment response. In the context of chronic hives, identifying reliable biomarkers can help clinicians assess disease progression, predict treatment outcomes, and tailor therapeutic interventions to individual patient needs. This section delves into the potential biomarkers used for disease monitoring in chronic hives and their implications for personalized treatment strategies.

Biomarkers for Disease Monitoring

1. Serum IgE Levels:

- Immunoglobulin E (IgE) plays a central role in allergic and immune-mediated responses and is implicated in the pathogenesis of chronic hives. Elevated serum IgE levels have been observed in some individuals with chronic hives, particularly those with allergic triggers or autoimmune mechanisms. Monitoring serum IgE levels over time can help clinicians assess disease activity and response to treatment, particularly in individuals receiving omalizumab therapy, which targets IgE.

2. Inflammatory Mediators:

- Various inflammatory mediators, including cytokines, chemokines, and histamine, contribute to the pathophysiology of chronic hives. Biomarkers such as interleukin-6 (IL-6), tumor necrosis factor-alpha (TNF-α), and C-reactive protein (CRP) have been associated with disease activity and severity in chronic hives. Monitoring changes in inflammatory mediator levels can provide insights into disease progression and response to anti-inflammatory therapies.

3. Autoantibodies:

- Autoantibodies targeting mast cell or basophil surface receptors, such as IgG anti-IgE autoantibodies or anti-FcεRI autoantibodies, are implicated in the pathogenesis of autoimmune-mediated chronic hives. Detection of autoantibodies in serum samples can help identify individuals with autoimmune mechanisms underlying their hives and guide treatment decisions, such as the use of immunomodulatory therapies or autologous serum therapy.

4. Basophil Activation Tests (BAT):

- Basophil activation tests (BAT) assess the responsiveness of basophils to stimuli, such as anti-IgE antibodies or allergens, by measuring cell surface marker expression (e.g., CD63, CD203c). BAT can help identify individuals with chronic hives who exhibit enhanced basophil activation in response to specific triggers, such as IgE-mediated or non-IgE-mediated mechanisms. Monitoring changes in basophil activation over time can provide valuable insights into disease activity and treatment response.

5. Skin Prick Testing (SPT) and Allergen-Specific IgE:

- Skin prick testing (SPT) and measurement of allergen-specific IgE levels can help identify allergic triggers in individuals with chronic hives. While not all cases of chronic hives are triggered by allergies, identifying and avoiding allergens can help reduce symptom severity and frequency in susceptible individuals. Monitoring changes in SPT results and allergen-specific IgE levels can guide allergen avoidance strategies and inform treatment decisions, such as allergen-specific immunotherapy.

6. Quality of Life Assessments:

- In addition to biological markers, assessments of quality of life, symptom severity, and psychosocial functioning are essential for evaluating disease burden and treatment outcomes in chronic hives. Patient-reported outcome measures (PROMs), such as the Chronic Urticaria Quality of Life Questionnaire (CU-Q2oL) or Urticaria Activity Score (UAS), provide valuable insights into the impact of hives on daily activities, emotional well-being, and overall quality of life. Monitoring changes in PROM scores can help clinicians assess treatment efficacy and patient satisfaction over time.

Conclusion:

Biomarkers play a critical role in disease monitoring and personalized treatment strategies for chronic hives. By identifying reliable biomarkers associated with disease activity, severity, and treatment response, clinicians can tailor therapeutic interventions to individual patient needs, optimize symptom control, and improve quality of life. From serum IgE levels and inflammatory mediators to autoantibodies, basophil activation tests, and allergen-specific markers, a comprehensive biomarker panel can provide valuable insights into the underlying mechanisms driving chronic hives and guide precision medicine approaches that enhance patient outcomes. As research continues to advance in the field of biomarker discovery and validation, the future holds promising opportunities for innovative biomarker-driven strategies that transform the management of chronic hives and improve patient care.

Exploring Novel Therapeutic Targets for Chronic Hives

Novel therapeutic targets offer promising avenues for the development of innovative treatments that address the underlying mechanisms driving chronic hives. By targeting specific pathways involved in immune dysregulation, inflammation, and histamine release, these novel therapies aim to provide more effective and tailored approaches to managing chronic hives. This section delves into potential novel therapeutic targets for chronic hives and their implications for future treatment strategies.

Novel Therapeutic Targets

1. Bruton's Tyrosine Kinase (BTK) Inhibitors:

- Bruton's tyrosine kinase (BTK) is a key regulator of B-cell signaling and activation, which plays a role in antibody production and immune responses. BTK inhibitors, such as ibrutinib and fenebrutinib, have shown efficacy in the treatment of B-cell malignancies and autoimmune disorders by modulating B-cell function and cytokine production. Given the involvement of B cells in the pathogenesis of chronic hives, BTK inhibitors represent a potential therapeutic target for modulating immune responses and reducing inflammation in refractory cases.

2. Prostaglandin D2 (PGD2) Receptor Antagonists:

- Prostaglandin D2 (PGD2) is a lipid mediator involved in allergic and inflammatory responses, including mast cell activation and eosinophil recruitment. PGD2 receptor antagonists, such as fevipiprant and timapiprant, have shown promise in the treatment of allergic diseases, such as asthma and allergic rhinitis. By blocking PGD2 signaling, these agents may help reduce mast cell activation and histamine release in chronic hives, providing symptomatic relief and improving disease control.

3. Spleen Tyrosine Kinase (SYK) Inhibitors:

- Spleen tyrosine kinase (SYK) is a signaling molecule involved in the activation of immune cells, including mast cells, basophils, and B cells. SYK inhibitors, such as fostamatinib, have demonstrated efficacy in the treatment of autoimmune and inflammatory conditions by inhibiting immune cell activation and cytokine production. In chronic hives, SYK inhibitors may modulate mast cell activation and downstream inflammatory responses, offering a novel therapeutic approach for symptom management and disease control.

4. CRTH2 Antagonists:

- Chemoattractant receptor-homologous molecule expressed on Th2 cells (CRTH2), also known as prostaglandin D2 receptor 2 (DP2), is a receptor expressed on Th2 cells and eosinophils involved in allergic inflammation. CRTH2 antagonists, such as setipiprant and OC000459, have demonstrated efficacy in the treatment of allergic diseases, including asthma and allergic rhinitis. By blocking CRTH2 signaling, these agents may attenuate eosinophilic inflammation and Th2-mediated immune responses in chronic hives, providing symptomatic relief and improving disease control.

5. Janus Kinase (JAK) Inhibitors:

- Janus kinase (JAK) inhibitors target the JAK-STAT signaling pathway, which plays a central role in cytokine signaling and immune cell activation. JAK inhibitors, such as ruxolitinib and tofacitinib, have shown efficacy in the treatment of autoimmune and inflammatory conditions, including rheumatoid arthritis and psoriasis. In chronic hives, JAK inhibitors may modulate cytokine production and immune cell activation, offering a novel therapeutic strategy for reducing inflammation and improving disease outcomes.

6. Neurokinin-1 (NK1) Receptor Antagonists:

- Neurokinin-1 (NK1) receptor antagonists, such as aprepitant and tradipitant, target the neurokinin-1 receptor, which is involved in neurogenic inflammation and pruritus. In chronic hives, neurogenic factors contribute to itch sensation and exacerbate inflammatory responses. NK1 receptor antagonists may attenuate neurogenic inflammation and pruritus, providing symptomatic relief and improving quality of life for individuals with chronic hives.

Conclusion:

Novel therapeutic targets hold great promise for the development of innovative treatments that address the underlying mechanisms driving chronic hives. From BTK inhibitors and PGD2 receptor antagonists to SYK inhibitors, CRTH2 antagonists, JAK inhibitors, and NK1 receptor antagonists, a diverse array of targeted therapies is emerging that aims to modulate immune responses, reduce inflammation, and alleviate symptoms in refractory cases of chronic hives. As research continues to advance in the field of novel therapeutic targets, the future holds exciting possibilities for personalized and precision medicine approaches that transform the management of chronic hives and improve patient outcomes.

Made in United States
Orlando, FL
16 July 2025

63038793R00075